Sarah Boston is a documentary film director and writer. Her publications include *Women Workers and the Trade Unions* and *Will, My Son*. She has a disorderly left breast which periodically causes lumps, pain, discharge and alarm. She has one daughter, her first child, Will, having died, and she lives in London.

Jill Louw is an SRN and worked for almost twenty years in nursing. She has breast cancer. It first appeared in 1980 and recurred in the same breast in 1985. She has three children, is Australian by birth and now lives in London.

Sarah Boston and Jill Louw

Disorderly Breasts

A guide to breast cancer, other breast disorders and their treatments

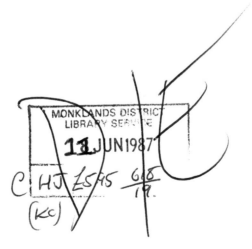

Camden Press

Published in 1987 by
Camden Press Ltd
43 Camden Passage, London N1 8EB, England

Set in Plantin 10½/12pt
by AKM Associates (UK) Limited
Ajmal House, Hayes Road, Southall, London
and printed and bound by
Richard Clay Ltd, Bungay, Suffolk

British Library Cataloguing in Publication Data
Boston, Sarah
    Disorderly breasts: a guide to breast
    cancer, other breast disorders and their
    treatments. — (Women's studies).
    1. Breast—Diseases
    I. Title   II. Louw, Jill   III. Series
    618.1'9   RG491

ISBN 0-948491-27-2

Contents

Acknowledgements

We should like to thank Dr Margaret Spittle, Consultant Radiotherapist at the Middlesex Hospital, for her professional advice, her personal support and for her careful checking of and helpful comments on the text. Likewise we should like to thank Ann Tait, Breast Cancer Nurse Counsellor at University College Hospital. Our thanks too go to all the women with breast disorders, cancerous and non-cancerous, who talked to us about their experiences and their feelings. Their contribution to this book, both in terms of the interviews we reproduce and in the greater understanding we gained from those women and the many more we talked to, is considerable.

For Emily, Charlotte, Daniel and Jessie

1. Introduction

The events leading up to the writing of this book started some years ago in a school playground. My daughter was in the same nursery class as Jill Louw's twin girls. Jill, however, was rarely to be seen at that period. Being curious I asked another woman about the twins' unseen mother. In hushed tones, almost a whisper, she told me, 'She has breast cancer.' Our conversation went little further than to comment, 'Poor woman.' My immediate reaction was to be filled with a sense of awe and fear: awe at the tragedy of the human condition made immediate by hearing of a woman with two small girls (I didn't know then she had an even smaller son), who carried what I assumed to be the death sentence of cancer. My fear was that that woman might be me. Immediately, as an almost unconscious physical reaction to my fear, I felt my breasts.

Sadly there was nothing untypical about that playground scene. Cancer is still talked about in hushed tones, because we feel threatened. Cancer is threatening to those with it and to those without it, and for women there is no more threatening a form of cancer than breast cancer. The fact that we could talk no further about Jill Louw was not just our ignorance of her case in particular but our ignorance of breast cancer in general. I gave myself a crash course in breast disorders not long after when I had my own breast 'scare', but it was to Jill that I turned when I wanted advice on who I should see for a second opinion. We got to talking about our own breast disorders and our discussions led me to write an article for the *Guardian* about Jill, her breast cancer and her refusal to have a mastectomy.

It was from the response to that article that the idea for the

1

book came. It was clear that many women, particularly those who have just had breast cancer diagnosed, are frightened and confused. Jill found herself answering the phone, writing letters and being asked in the street and the playground for advice and support. It was evident women needed information, support and someone to whom they could talk about their experiences.

Thus this book started out of two women's experiences, one of breast cancer, the other of a non-cancerous breast disorder, and was provoked into being by the experience of many others. From the outset we therefore decided that women's actual experience of breast disorders, much ignored, should form an integral part of the book. It was both our stepping-off point and our point of referral. We talked to many women who have or have had breast disorders and include some of their case histories in the book. Jill's own case history had, even during the researching and writing of this book, to be updated. For in 1985, five years after the removal of her primary cancerous tumour, she developed a recurrence in the same breast. Personal experience of breast cancer was thus a continuing backdrop to our work.

Talking to other women was also important to us, for it was through our discussions and interviews that we learned what women would like to know, how they feel, how they would like to be treated, and what follow-up support they would appreciate.

Since the majority of women in Britain with breast disorders are most likely to be treated by orthodox medical practitioners working in the National Health Service, the main body of this book is based on that system and the treatment it offers. However, we also recognize that most patients have a more open mind about different medical systems than those who practise those systems. Few women with breast cancer opt entirely for orthodox medicine or alternative medicine. The more common pattern is for patients to take a bit from both, hedging their bets and exercising their right to choose. Usually women have some form of orthodox primary treatment and then look elsewhere for other preventive treatments. So women have surgery and then go on the Bristol diet, or they take the drug Tamoxifen and swallow vitamin pills. They try to attack cancerous growths through the power of their mind by the visualization technique while also taking drugs to attack the growth. Doctors treat women's sick bodies, but increasingly the women look elsewhere, to self-help and support groups, for their mental health. This search for the best possible treatment arises from the fact that there is no known cure for breast cancer. There are only a variety of treatments. About those treatments there is a wide variety of opinion. Within orthodox medicine, debate ranges over the benefits of the four forms of treatment – surgery, radiotherapy, chemotherapy and hormone therapy. There have been trials about different forms of treatment and different combinations of treatment, and more trials are underway. There is much argument about the findings of those trials already conducted. Not only is there wide disagreement about treatments, there is an equally wide range of opinion about the possible causes of breast cancer. It is not surprising that patients who are caught up in all this are confused.

Because of the lack of any known cure it is of particular importance that whatever the treatment a woman should agree to it voluntarily, without pressure, having being informed of its benefits and its risks. This book above all is about informed consent. It is about the patient's right to choose and the realization that choice cannot be exercised in a state of ignorance and fear. Women have much to offer each other in the support and strength gained through shared experience. From being frightened, ignorant and powerless individuals, we can become an informed group, who with, we hope, the help of the professionals, can begin to win the war against breast cancer.

Sarah Boston

2. Finding something wrong

It was late April, one morning at half past seven. I can tell you exactly where I was standing. I discovered this lump right on the side of my breast quite close to where it joins the wall of the body.

(Hazel)

As I was painting the kitchen I became convinced my left nipple was wet. I was so convinced that I took off my sweater and there on my bra was a small wet patch.

(Sarah)

I first found a lump about the size of my little finger nail. I was on holiday. I just felt this lump round there on the right side near the armpit. I thought, No, there's not. I'd actually had a lump before on my left breast when I was about 21 and had that removed at the Charing Cross Hospital, and in fact that was a small cyst. So I'd been through it before, but I think I felt differently this time. I think I felt much more frightened. All day long I kept feeling and thinking, Is it there? No it's not. Yes it is.

(Jenny)

In the absence of any systematic examination and screening system for breast disorders, most symptoms are found by women themselves, often quite by chance. Regular breast self-examination has not yet become a way of life for women, particularly those in the high risk group, those from 35 to 55 years of age. Later in this book we will look at the techniques and

4

benefits of examining one's own breasts and of other screening methods. Here the important thing that women should know and take mental note of are the signs that something is wrong with their breast or breasts.

A lump is the best-known symptom and the one that causes most fear. Eighty per cent of lumps in the breast are not cancerous, but that fact is of no reassurance to a woman on first finding one. Other symptoms can also be signs of cancer, but much more frequently they are signs of some other, non-cancerous breast disorder. The breasts, like the other parts of a woman's reproductive system, are vulnerable to disease and disorder. Any of the following symptoms indicate that something is amiss with the breast and on observing one or more of them a woman should take action. Ignoring them and hoping that they will go away could be a very dangerous path to take.

In general the symptoms to act upon are any change in or on the breast, the nipple, the area around the breast including the armpit, the upper arm and the area of chest above the breast. Pain in any of those areas should not be ignored. The following is a checklist of symptoms:

1. The breast. Any change in the size or shape of the breast, either by one breast getting larger or smaller and harder. Any flattening, bulging, dimpling, puckering of the skin or change in the skin surface, especially if the skin begins to look like the skin of an orange. Veins standing out more than usual and, of course, any lumps.

2. The nipple. Any change in the size, shape or position of the nipple, especially if it shows sign of inverting, flattening or dimpling. Discharge from the nipple, whether containing blood or not, and any change in the brown skin surrounding the nipple (the areola), particularly if the skin appears to be ulcerous, to have eczema or spots.

3. The armpit and upper arm. As with the breast, any change should be acted upon. Particular attention should be paid to any swelling of the upper arm or the armpit.

4. *The chest wall above the breast*. Any swelling should also be acted upon, as well as any change in the skin surface.
5. *Moles*. Note should be taken of any moles on the breast, chest, upper arm and neck area, and any change in size or colour should be investigated.
6. *Pain*. Although common wisdom is that pain is not a sign of cancer, at least in its earliest stages, pain should not be ignored. Recent research has shown that in a minority of cases, some 10 per cent, women diagnosed as having breast cancer had pain as one of their symptoms.

The above list seems alarming and might cause women to think they should spend at least part of every day scrutinizing themselves for any minute change. It may have the reverse effect and cause some women to be so frightened of what they might find that they will never look at or feel their breasts. By the end of the book we hope women will have less fear, feel more in control and better equipped to confront their own body.

3. First visit

I plucked up courage and went and saw Dr W., the student doctor down there, and he examined me and he just didn't seem to have a clue, sort of went, 'Oh yeah, when did you first feel the lump?' and all the rest of it. Then he said, 'Do you mind if I get a second opinion on this?' So he left me sitting there and called Dr X. He examined me and asked me the same questions. He prodded around and examined me again and said, 'Right. Put your bra and blouse back on again.' I was just sitting there while they were discussing me.

(Ann)

I discovered a lump in my left breast and went to my doctor after about three or four months. She felt the breast and she said, 'No, it just feels like a lumpy breast to me. If it still bothers you, come back.' I went away and thought, 'That's all right, fine, forget about it', because I didn't really want to know about it.

(Jo)

All books and advisory pamphlets on breast disorders tell women to go *straight away* to their doctor on finding any of the symptoms described in Chapter 1. Despite this, many women delay for weeks, months and even years before taking the advice. They usually delay nowadays not because of ignorance but because of fear: fear that their symptom is that of cancer, a life-threatening disease, and fear that it is *breast* cancer, which many women assume will mean, if treated, the loss of a breast

7

(mastectomy) and thus a loss of identity as women. It is understandable that faced with the prospect of mutilating surgery and the threat to their very existence some women are paralysed with fear. Most women will discover on investigation that their symptoms are not cancerous and that going straight away to a doctor is the speediest route to ending sleepless nights and days of fear. For the few who find that their symptoms are those of cancer, going to a doctor might not only avert death but might also avert mastectomy. There is no doubt that the earlier cancer is detected the better the chances are of a cure. Also the earlier the detection the greater the chances are that a woman will not be pressurized into having a mastectomy. More surgeons are now prepared to treat small tumours with the removal of the lump only (a lumpectomy), with or without additional treatment involving radiotherapy, chemotherapy and hormone therapy – all discussed in later sections of the book.

Whatever the course of treatment a woman chooses, including opting for alternative medicine or seeking complementary treatment, the earlier she acts the better. Going straight away for advice is of crucial importance, although it is not always as easy to do as it is to recommend. Sensitivity to the fact that many women find it difficult to pluck up courage to go to a doctor led to the setting up in some cities of 'walk-in' clinics attached to hospitals where women with symptoms of breast disorders may, without having made an appointment, just walk in. It was hoped that such clinics would encourage women not to put off diagnosis and treatment. Being able just to walk in removes the stress of having to make an appointment. It also means that the first examination is much more likely to be carried out by a woman in a clinic where they are experienced in breast examination and are more sympathetic to women's anxieties. Walk-in clinics are few and far between and in their absence a woman might prefer her initial examination to be at a 'Well Woman' clinic than by a general practitioner. Most 'Well Woman' clinics routinely examine the breasts of women already attending the clinic, but there is no reason why a woman cannot make an appointment specifically for this. As with the 'walk-in' clinics, women might well find a 'Well Woman' clinic less intimidating than going to their general practitioners.

Many women are neither close to a 'walk-in' clinic nor a 'Well Woman' clinic and they must first go to a general practitioner. Some have no hesitation in making their first appointment, but others do and for them that first visit can be a major ordeal. Asking to see a woman doctor in a practice can make it less stressful, though it does not follow that women doctors, by virtue of their sex alone, are more sympathetic. Their training is the same as that of their male colleagues in the profession. A quick bit of 'consumer research', asking other people who use the same practice, can help in finding out which doctor is likely to be the most sympathetic and prepared to listen as well as to advise.

It has to be remembered that despite their training general practitioners have relatively little daily experience of examining patients with possible breast cancer. Dr Dennis Wang from the Imperial Cancer Research Fund estimated that a general practitioner with an average list of 2,500 patients would have about 600 women on that list at risk. Of that 600 the general practitioner would see only six new patients with breast cancer in every 10 years of practice. Women should bear that in mind when first seeing their general practitioner, especially if she or he is dismissive, saying, 'There is nothing to worry about.' For example, one woman was told by her general practitioner, when she went to see him about a discharge from one nipple, that she was just fantasizing because she really wanted another child. She had had four children and by mutual consent her husband had had a vasectomy. However, general practitioners are much less dismissive than in the past. They are much more likely to refer women to hospitals for further investigation than to pat them on the heads and say, 'Go home, don't worry.'

At the first visit to a general practitioner or to a clinic the procedure will be the same. Having told the doctor why you have come, you will be asked to strip to the waist. The doctor will then stand back and look at you. Given our culture and its emphasis

9

on breasts as sex objects and symbols, it is hard to stand there having your breasts scrutinized and not to feel embarrassed, let alone afraid of what the doctor might see. Also, it is hard to cope with the fact that the doctor is not looking at your sex symbols but she, or more frequently he, is looking to see if one or both of your breasts show any of the signs of abnormality or difference listed in Chapter 1. The doctor will then ask you to lie down and she or he will feel your breasts and the area around them, including the underarm. The medical term for this process of feeling is 'palpation'. A doctor unfamiliar with the everyday usage of the English language might say, 'I am now going to palpate your breasts', but most doctors are more likely to say, 'I am now going to feel your breasts.' Perhaps the most courteous approach would be for the doctor to say 'May I now feel your breasts', and explain the necessity for doing so.

After examining you, the caring doctor should ask if you have any questions, what your worries are and what your family history is in relation to breast disorders. The experience of women during their first visit to a general practitioner reveals that doctors all too rarely take the time to explain what they are doing and why, to ask questions or to take the time to listen to their patients. Dr Peter Maguire, who studied the psychiatric problems of women with breast cancer, advises general practitioners, who after all have the long-term care of the patient, to establish the basis of a caring and trusting relationship from the outset. He advises general practitioners to 'be honest, maintain hope and be solicitous of their patients' feelings.' His research has shown that the attitudes of those members of the medical profession who treat women with breast cancer is a crucial element in the extent to which a woman is able to cope with and confront her disease.

Since all general practitioners all too rarely offer such human care women should try, as far as they are able, to demand it. Such demands in themselves create change. An American doctor, Dr Allan H Bruckheim, who trains family physicians in a New Jersey hospital, claims that patients by their questioning of doctors' attitudes have forced change. In the *Sunday Times* of

21 April 1985 he was quoted as saying of doctors, 'We can no longer have the autocratic, chauvinistic and paternalistic doctor that was common until a decade ago. It's not good enough to say, "I'll cure you or I'll cut it out".' American doctors have realized that patients go 'doctor-shopping', the effect of which has been to make doctors much more responsive to the needs of their patients. Despite the difference of systems, there is nothing to stop the National Health patient going 'doctor-shopping' too. It is a question that will be dealt with again in this book.

Usually the general practitioner, after examining you and often without any further discussion, will then refer you for further investigations at a breast unit in a hospital. This referral is done, more often then not, in the terms 'I don't think it is anything to worry about but . . .' In terms of statistics the doctor is right, but in terms of human emotion a woman is almost certainly going to worry. Few doctors, having suggested the need to refer a woman to a hospital consultant, will take the time or trouble to explain what kind of 'further investigations' are likely to be done. Any woman would be wise to accept referral if only to have the opportunity of accurate diagnosis. Alternative medicine has not yet developed accurate diagnostic methods. Women equally should not rest assured by the doctor telling her, 'There is nothing to worry about.' While it may be, almost certainly is, what a woman wants to hear, it isn't necessarily in her best interests to hear it. In general a woman with any of the symptoms listed in Chapter 1 should insist to her doctor that she be referred for further investigations. It is not only right, but the figures for breast cancer, that one woman in sixteen gets it, should make any doctor or woman be vigilant and never take such symptoms lightly. If you have any of those symptoms you are not a neurotic woman but a woman with symptoms of a breast disorder that just might be cancer.

4. First referral

I went back a week later, exactly the same and the GP said, 'Well, it's possibly a cyst. We'll send you along to a great friend of mine, Mr X at the Hospital. You just go along and make sure it's all right.

(Hazel)

Then he said, 'I think you should see our breast surgeon, Dr Y.' Well, then I started shaking, as soon as he said surgeon, well, I mean imagine someone with a knife, ready there. The GP said to me, 'Don't worry, she's not going to cut it off yet.' That was the exact words to me.

(Ann)

While women should accept, or even demand, referral to a consultant for further investigations and diagnosis, to whom one is referred, and where, is of crucial importance. Where one is referred to is crucial, because hospitals offer different services and have differing attitudes towards the treatment, both medical and psychological, of women with breast disorders. Even more important is to whom one is referred, since the treatment offered and the attitudes towards patients stem mainly from those at the top – the consultants.

Surgeons deal with breast cancer in British hospitals and most women accept the surgeon to whom they are referred by their GP. They take on your case and only through them might your case be discussed with other specialists within orthodox medicine. It is hardly surprising that since surgeons are the people who deal with breast disorders surgery has been the main form of treatment. Increasingly treatment of breast disorders in general, and in particular breast cancer, has become much more complex than simple surgery. It now often involves specialists with other skills besides those of surgery and this has led to the formation of breast units. Despite the formation in some hospitals of these units, a woman's first appointment at a breast clinic will be with a surgeon or one of his or her team. With the emergence of breast units, the logical development would seem to be the training of breast specialists, who would have less of an investment in surgery as the prime or only form of treatment and be more open to discussion both with professional colleagues and with patients – the best combination of known treatments for that particular case.

For the time being, however, you will be referred to a general surgeon who also deals with breast cases. Most GPs will refer you to the surgeon they know of or to the one at the nearest breast unit. You can ask to be referred to the person of your choice. While it is your right to do so, and sometimes a GP will ask you if you have a preference, most women do not have the information with which to exercise their right or even to express a preference. Getting that information is not easy if it is not given by the GP. If you are accepting the referral of your GP's choice, it would be wise to ask your GP whether he or she knows what the attitude and practices are of the surgeon you are being sent to see.

Surgeon-shopping is even harder than doctor-shopping. There is no 'Good Breast Clinic Guide' on a par with the *Good Birth Guide*. It is hard to find what the attitude of different surgeons is, apart from the one or two who have 'gone public' and written books or been interviewed on the subject. In making a choice it would help patients if hospitals, like schools, publicly stated what their policies are, but hospitals make no such public statement. They work on the assumption that the treatment they offer is of the best possible standard, affected only by limitations on their ability to spend money and the limitations of medical knowledge. In relation to breast cancer the limitations of medical knowledge are considerable. Since the Second World

War, despite advances in medicine in other areas, there has been no reduction in the number of deaths from breast cancer. It continues to be the cause of the highest number of deaths among women between 35 and 55 – 5,000 women die from it every year in the United Kingdom. There has also been a slight increase in the incidence of breast cancer, but it is hard to know whether that is due to greater awareness and to screening facilities or to other factors. Fortunately the future for women looks just a little brighter. While no single breakthrough has been made in the treatment or cure of breast cancer, recent research and trials are showing evidence that more women can be cured – that is, either they can live out their life without a recurrence, or if cancer recurs then it can be controlled.

Given the current state of medical knowledge and the fact that surgeons are still quite divided in their beliefs about the best possible form of treatment for women with breast cancer, it is hardly surprising that women should want to go surgeon-shopping. Whilst some women welcome decisions being made for them and are happy to accept that 'doctor knows best', an increasing number of women expect to be treated as intelligent and sentient human beings. They expect a consultation with a 'consultant' to be a two-way interchange. Finding a surgeon with whom one can communicate and in whom one has confidence may well be a question of trial and error, although when so much is at stake minimizing the chance of error is important. If a GP cannot help then the best course is to ask other women. Women who have had experience of breast disorders are most likely to be found through one of the organizations listed at the end of this book.

The advantage of going to a GP for your first visit rather than to a walk-in clinic attached to a hospital is that you can exercise a choice. If you go to a walk-in clinic you will, if necessary, automatically be referred to the surgeon or one of his or her team at that hospital. Of course for many women they have no choice or very little choice. Choice is the luxury of those who live in the big city areas. Those women outside big cities will be referred to the nearest hospital that treats breast disorders.

On referral you will be given a sealed letter by your GP to take to the hospital with you. Most of us rush home and open the letter. New electric kettles that cut off at boiling point make steaming letters open difficult so the other way is to open it, buy another brown envelope and re-seal it. On the whole GPs' letters of referral reveal very little, merely giving the reason, usually in illegible handwriting, for referral. On the whole GPs don't commit themselves to a diagnostic opinion. It is relatively easy to gather this tiny bit of information sent by the GP to the consultant. Later it becomes much harder, indeed it can be a battle, to find out which of your personal records the hospital keeps.

The question of 'open medical records' – open to the patient concerned – is a hot one. Most of the medical profession are against opening the files to patients. Most patients want to see the files. The medical profession argue that some patients 'can't take' certain kinds of information. Most patients argue that they find fear and suspicion more terrifying than the truth. While there may be a justifiable concern that in a few cases information in the files might seriously disturb a patient, the concern of patients is not so much the medical information and records contained in the files but the medical profession's moral comments. On files go phrases like 'This patient is hysterical, neurotic, difficult and aggressive.' They include words which do not record clinical information but describe a doctor's feelings about a patient's behaviour. Many women keep a brave face and a stiff upper lip in front of consultants for fear that they will be seen as 'hysterical' and that this perception will go on file. Likewise patients fear questioning a doctor's opinion precisely because such questioning will be interpreted as being 'a difficult patient'. Thus labelled, patients fear it may well affect their subsequent treatment.

This fear is not without reason. Des Wilson, arguing in the *Observer* of 8 September 1985 for the right of each individual to have access to records and files kept about them, wrote:

> In a recent article for the medical journal *Pulse*, a doctor
> from Aberdeen defended secrecy of medical records. 'All

15

GPs, I imagine, have in moments of pique written unfair and maybe even untrue things about troublesome patients on their record. Are patients to have free access to read these?' In these two sentences he unintentionally demonstrated why it is essential that we *do* have access to, and the opportunity to correct, files kept about ourselves.

Medicine, like so many other aspects of British life, is highly secretive. A few doctors have voluntarily opened their files to their patients and more and more patients are demanding that their files be opened. Until such time as patients have the legal right to see their medical records, all one can do is to ask. One can at least ask to check that the records are accurate. Mistakes have been made.

While the records remain closed, the small brown envelope from your GP to the hospital can be opened. Clutching it, and with the knowledge of its contents, a woman referred to a hospital will, anxious if not terrified, go for her first visit. There her breast disorder will be diagnosed.

5. Diagnosis

Clinical examination

I heard (from the hospital) about three weeks later and I
went and again it was another week. I saw the registrar. He
was very pleasant and he talked about my job and mauled
it around and moved it a lot and said, 'Well, it's not very
stuck to the wall. It's not very stuck. It's probably all right,
but . . .' and very casually he said, 'I think we'll just have
you in for a look.'

(Hazel)

A week later I got an appointment for the following week. I
went down and saw a young doctor down there. He
examined me and asked the same questions again. Why
hadn't I gone sooner? Was I worried about it? And then he
said, 'I don't think it is anything to worry about, but I'm
going to book you in for a mammogram.' He didn't explain
what a mammogram was. I hadn't a clue what he was
talking about.

(Ann)

Having been told to go *straight away* without *delay* to your GP
on finding any symptoms, you will have to wait before going to
hospital for your first out-patients appointment. Most hospitals,
except the walk-in clinics, have a breast clinic once a week. The
average delay between GP and out-patients seems to be about
two weeks. Having waited to go to the hospital, when you get
there you will almost certainly have to wait, minutes or hours,

17

again. Getting a friend or partner to go with you can help to minimize the stress and make the waiting time seem shorter. Unfortunately many women feel that 'it', the fear that what they have may be breast cancer, is something they cannot talk about, not even to their husband, partner or closest friend. Being able to break the silence is important and can be very helpful. In general it is better to talk to somebody than to nobody. Talking about 'it' is something to which we shall return later, particularly in relation to nurse counsellors.

On seeing the surgeon or one of his or her team at the hospital, the procedure will initially be the same as at the first visit to the GP. You will be asked to strip to the waist and to sit. When you have done so you will first be looked at and then asked to lie down to have both your breasts and the area around them felt. Questions will be asked of your symptoms, how long you have had them, your family medical history and your own personal medical history.

If one of your symptoms is a lump the doctor will feel to see whether it is hard or soft, mobile or fixed, and will ask whether or not it is tender. The doctor will also be trying to feel whether the lump is a distinct one as opposed to being part of a general lumpiness in the breast. 'Lumpy breasts', a somewhat unflattering description of the feel of some women's breasts, have different causes but are rarely cancerous. The underarm area will also be carefully felt to see if there is any swelling. Doctors can get a fair indication of the nature of the disease from the feel and location of the lump, but they will always do further tests to confirm their initial diagnosis.

If discharge is one of your symptoms you will be asked to describe the discharge: the colour of it, particularly whether it is clear or bloodstained; whether it is a thick liquid or thin; and, if possible, whether the discharge is from one duct on one nipple or from many ducts on one or both nipples. You will then be asked to try to express some discharge from one or both nipples. Anyone who has expressed breast milk at least they will know how to try to express discharge. For those who haven't, the usual technique is to use the thumb and forefinger and with light

18

pressure slowly stroke the nipple from outside of the brown area around the nipple (the areola) inwards to the nipple. However, even for those experienced in the art of expressing milk, trying to express a discharge when you are nervous, being watched and probably cold, so that your nipple goes hard, is quite a daunting task. If you are too daunted or unable to do it, then it is worth asking if you might retire to another room with a nurse where you can try to do it in your own time. Assuming you manage to express even a droplet it will be collected and sent to the laboratory for analysis. Such analysis is important since it can provide vital evidence in diagnosing your breast disorder.

However confident the consultant is in his or her diagnosis, you will almost certainly be sent for a mammogram. This usually means making another appointment at the hospital – and another period of waiting. Even patients for whom the doctor requires a biopsy usually also have a mammogram.

Mammogram

I went to the hospital about two weeks later, for a mammogram, which is . . . well, I didn't like that in the least. It was done by a woman. She was OK. She explained what she was going to do to me. She did the mammogram and said, 'We'll find out the results and we'll give you an appointment for another week's time.'

(Ann)

A mammogram was taken and right from the beginning I decided that I was going to be in control, so I took my camera and asked the woman who did the mammogram if I could take a photograph of the mammogram being done. She said she didn't think it was a very good idea and then she said, 'Oh yes, I'll take it for you.' I said, 'I just want it as a record', and she said, 'Don't tell anyone it was taken here, because I could get into trouble.' So right from the beginning I was asking questions but not asking medical questions. It was like a game.

(Jo)

A mammogram is a form of X-ray using radiation. It is argued that new 'low-dose' mammography using half a rad on the skin exposed is safe. This amount being approximately one-hundredth of that previously used. So if you are having a mammogram it is worth checking that you are being X-rayed with new 'low-dose' machines. It is claimed that these new low-dose mammograms expose the patient to unharmful doses of radiation, although there are those who maintain that any exposure to radiation is potentially harmful.

The advantage of mammography is that it can detect tumours (not necessarily malignant ones) which are under two centimetres and which therefore cannot be detected by clinical examination. In brief it can show up those lumps that are too small to be felt. The exposure of a woman to the level of radiation received in a single low-dose mammogram is not so much questioned as the use of mammography as a screening device in which case women would be or are exposed to a culminative amount of radiation. Later we shall discuss in detail the debate over mammography as a screening device and the use of other means of obtaining an image or picture of the inside of the breast.

The almost routine use of mammography as a diagnostic tool, except for certain cases, in some breast clinics is also questioned. Patients with a definite lump, 'a discrete palpable lump' as it is described by doctors, should be referred immediately for a biopsy, as a mammogram can only confirm the existence of a lump. All too frequently women find that after the mammogram they are told, 'All it shows is you've got a lump', which most of them knew in the first place. Mammography can help in diagnosis when the symptoms are less definite. It can help in trying to distinguish between general lumpiness and a possibly more serious lump which can not be felt. In patients with other symptoms such as discharge and pain it can help to reassure the doctor that no more sinister unfelt lump is in the breast. A woman referred for a mammogram would be wise to ask whether it is really necessary.

Besides the risk of exposure to radiation, most women find having a mammogram a demeaning, uncomfortable and sometimes painful experience. In order to X-ray the breast you are asked to strip to the waist and two X-rays of each breast are taken. In order to X-ray the breast, it is first laid out flat on a metal plate and a second metal plate is brought down horizontally on to the first so that your breast is sandwiched in-between. It seems that only women with medium-sized breasts come out of the experience complaining of it being merely 'uncomfortable'. The second X-ray is taken with your breast sandwiched between the metal plates vertically. The procedure is then repeated on the other breast. For most women with particularly large or small breasts sandwiching them is difficult and can leave the breasts bruised.

After the mammogram, once again you will have to wait for another appointment to get the results. If the mammogram confirms the existence of a lump, or detects a lump not previously detected, then the surgeon will want to make a further investigation to decide whether the lump is cancerous or not and then to decide what form of treatment may be appropriate. There continues to be division over which is the best way to get that crucial further piece of information. The old method still used by some surgeons is 'the frozen section', or excisional, biopsy, and certain surgeons still use it sometimes. The new method used increasingly is the 'needle biopsy'.

Biopsy

> So then I saw the doctor and he said, 'We're not absolutely certain what's there, so we'll have to do a needle biopsy this morning. Anyway, the lump is quite big, so you'll probably have to go into hospital and have it removed. At the time you get into hospital they'll know whether it is cancer or not.'
>
> (Jo)

> I had the biopsy and I came round quite quickly and I had this plaster across here [indicating the left side of her left breast]. That night my family came to see me. All that day

21

and the next day I was waiting, waiting, waiting. All
Tuesday, I kept seeing this houseman and saying,
'Anything?' 'No,' he said. 'Anything?' 'No.' 'Anything?'
'No.'

(Hazel)

Before I had the biopsy they told me. They obviously knew
what it was, or were pretty certain, because I think there
were lumps under the arm. They felt that there was
something under this arm as well. I didn't know it was
malignant until I came out, until after, in and out. But I
had said to them they could take the breast off if . . .

(Gladys)

A biopsy is the name of a process in which a small amount of
tissue from a suspicious lump is removed. The tissue is then sent
to a laboratory for analysis by a pathologist. There are various
ways in which a biopsy can be done. Until very recently it was
almost always done under general anaesthetic and called an
excisional biopsy, a small cut would be made and tissue
removed. More recently an increasing number of biopsies are
done in out-patients departments or the patient may be
admitted to a day ward. One type of out-patient biopsy is done
using a local anaesthetic. Into the anaesthetized area a small stab
incision is made so that the cutting needle may be inserted in
order to remove some tissue. Another method is called fine
needle aspiration. As its name suggests a fine needle is inserted
into the lump and a small amount of tissue, usually only a cluster
of cells but enough for analysis, is sucked out. The choice of
which type of biopsy to perform on a patient is in most cases
made on the basis of the preference of the surgeon and the skills
of those in the breast clinic team. Sometimes the nature and
position of the lump indicates which type of biopsy is needed.

Excisional biopsy
There are very few cases in which a biopsy under a general
anaesthetic is necessary. Such biopsies appear to be done now

more in the interests of the surgeon than of the patient, except in those few cases where needle sampling and other diagnostic methods have been inconclusive and there remains doubt. The biopsy itself performed under general anaesthetic has been of less concern to women than the reasons why it was and still is done. Tissue removed by excision is fast frozen and rushed to a laboratory while the patient is still anaesthetized.

Once the results have come back from the laboratory, the surgeon will decide whether or not to operate further. It is a situation with which women for decades have had to cope. They are put to sleep not knowing whether they will wake up with one breast or two. The nightmare of such a situation was, and in some hospitals still is, very real. It seems that the only reason why this practice continues is that surgeons, in the interests of productivity, immediately perform any surgery they think necessary while they have the patient on the table. After all, the patient has signed a consent form, but true consent must necessarily be based on information. During an excision biopsy only the surgeon has the information on the frozen section; the patient is unconscious. It is hardly surprising that more and more women are saying that even if a frozen section is the only diagnostic method offered, then they will refuse to consent to further surgery unless they are allowed to be woken from the anaesthetic and given time to consider and to discuss different forms of treatment. The question of informed consent is something we shall return to many times throughout this book.

There is absolutely no medical reason why a patient should not be allowed to regain consciousness and be given plenty of time to consider which course of action she would like to take. It is curious that from first referral to a hospital to admission for a biopsy many weeks can pass in waiting for appointments, yet it is argued that if the frozen section reveals that the tumour is cancerous then it is crucial, a life and death issue, that surgery is immediately performed. The argument doesn't hold. While submitting someone to two anaesthetics in a short period of time is more hazardous than merely having one, the hazard is small compared to the long-term effect on many women of feeling unable to decide for themselves whether or not to have surgery. Equally important, the information based on a frozen section that can be given speedily is limited. In the time available the surgeon can only be told whether or not the tumour is cancerous. Further analysis, which could be important in choosing treatment, cannot be gathered.

One can only assume that surgeons don't wake patients up to consult with them because in the interests of efficiency and in keeping the production line moving it is cheaper and quicker to do everything at once. Such a procedure also protects the surgeon from having to discuss the disease, to answer questions, to confront the patient's distress and possibly to deal with a patient who rejects the treatment the surgeon thinks is in their best interest.

If your surgeon suggests an excision biopsy, first make sure it *is* the only form of biopsy that can be performed on your particular lump. Read the consent form *very, very* carefully and don't sign it if you have the slightest question until it has been answered to your satisfaction. Also *check* the consent form very carefully. Check that no errors have been made. More than one woman has found instructions about the wrong breast written down on the form.

Needle biopsy
There are two basic methods of out-patient needle biopsy. Some surgeons claim that cutting needle biopsy is the best method, whilst others argue for fine needle aspiration. The advantage of both is that they can be done in an out-patients clinic on the patient's first visit, thus speeding up the process and rendering unnecessary a general anaesthetic for diagnostic purposes.

Theoretically the cutting needle biopsy should not hurt if adequate local anaesthetic has been given. This is given by injection with a fine needle around the area of the lump. Since the anaesthetic may not penetrate the lump, the area from which the tissue is taken, the process may be uncomfortable or even painful, although it should be a brief pain. Following the biopsy the small cut will probably require a stitch or two.

24

When you return to out-patients for the removal of your stitches, the results of the biopsy will be given to you. Being an out-patient makes the discussion with the doctors and with friends and family about different forms of treatment much more possible.

It was precisely for that reason that some centres have pioneered fine needle aspirations. For some time women with cysts have had their cysts aspirated by needle biopsy. It involves sticking the needle into the cyst and drawing off the fluid from inside, thus giving almost immediate relief from pain. For safety, some of that fluid is sent for analysis. Since most lumps are not cancerous the process not only gives women with cysts physical relief from the tenderness and/or pain of a cyst but gives them mental relief and reassurance. In the early stages surgeons were reluctant to use needle biopsy for cancer diagnosis as it was found not to be as accurate as the frozen section method. However, places which have pioneered fine needle biopsy and who have developed their techniques now find that they get a very high rate of accuracy. In Edinburgh in particular, surgeons have performed needle biopsies for some time and realized that in skilled hands only a few cases required surgery for a definitive diagnosis. In 1983 they reported to the *Lancet*, 'Fine needle aspiration cytology can achieve a definitive diagnosis in over 90% of carcinomas without recourse to surgery, so diagnosis and treatment options can be discussed with the patient pre-operatively.'

Not only can this type of biopsy be done at the first visit to an out-patients clinic, but since analysis is of a few cells only, diagnosis can be made in minutes. The terrible waiting period is thus reduced to a short period in the clinic during one's first out-patient visit.

It is interesting to note that one of the main reasons for use of fine needle biopsy, as argued in the *Lancet*, is that 'treatment options' can be discussed. In other words, you won't be put to sleep not knowing how you will wake up. You have time to discuss forms of treatment with the surgeon. You have time to feel that you can make your own decision about your own body.

Some women feel they have made that decision in their minds before even getting the results, but many have not. But while this form of biopsy gives scope for discussion of treatment options, that discussion does not always take place. Many surgeons still tell you what form of treatment they will give you. But you at least are awake, conscious, and have time to raise questions.

Having by one means or another diagnosed your disorder, the surgeon will then suggest the form of treatment he or she thinks best. It is at this point that 'informed consent' becomes a crucial issue.

6. Informed consent

Finally he found this note and then got a pen out of his
pocket and said, 'That's the breast that is coming off', and
put a cross on the breast.

(Jo)

'Yes, it is bad news.' It was as blunt as that. He then
removed the stitches and whilst he was doing so told me
that I could be re-admitted on Easter Monday for a
mastectomy on the Tuesday. I was assured it was very
simple surgery and that I would be home on the following
Friday.

(Jill)

He's a particular surgeon who for women in their thirties,
who very much wants them to have oopherectomies
(removal of the ovaries) following a mastectomy. He doesn't
give you much time to breathe, because one week it's
mastectomy and the following week it's the oopherectomy.

(Jenny)

The newscaster on the BBC Nine O'clock News on 21 February
1985, reporting a decision of the Law Lords, said that it was
'something of a trend' for patients to ask for more information
from the doctors treating them. It was put as though such a
quest for information was like the flavour of the season and one
which, to the satisfaction of some in the medical profession,
would, like the seasons, change. The Law Lords did their best to
defend the status quo and halt the trend. In their ruling on the

case of Mrs Amy Sidaway who claimed that she would never have agreed to an operation had she been informed that there was a risk of her being left partially paralysed, they ruled that the doctor was not obliged to inform her of all the potential risks. Lord Diplock said,

> The only effect that mention of risks can have on the patient's mind, if it has any at all, can be in the direction of deterring the patient from undergoing the treatment which in the expert opinion of the doctor it is in the patient's interests to undergo.

While the Law Lords did not support Mrs Sidaway, Lord Scarman did use the opportunity to indicate that he thought the doctrine of 'informed consent', as practised in some parts of the USA, should be introduced into Britain.

Not surprisingly, the treatment of women with breast cancer was one of the central areas of concern that led to demands for the doctrine of informed consent to be legislated for in some states.

In the state of Massachusetts there is now a state law that not only deals with patients' rights in general, but has a specific amendment which singles out breast cancer. It stipulates that 'in the case of a patient suffering from any form of breast cancer, the patient has the right to complete information on all alternative treatments which are medically viable'. Commenting on that clause, Judy Norsigian, one of the authors of *Our Bodies Ourselves: A Health Book By and For Women*, the Boston Women's Health Collective book (London: Allen Lane, 1978), told the *Family Practice News*,

> 'To most surgeons, alternative forms of treatment means alternative forms of surgery. Now, if a physician does not discuss chemotherapy, radiotherapy and surgery, he would be breaking the law, not just ethical practice.'

Increasingly women wish to know about alternative and

complementary forms of medicine. Unfortunately, since the practitioners of alternative and orthodox medicine are often more or less in two warring camps, each side is unlikely to discuss possible forms of treatment advocated by the other.

The demand for informed consent, particularly in relation to breast cancer, has no doubt arisen from the fact that in the USA mastectomy was and largely still is the routine treatment for breast cancer. Indeed, some surgeons have gone so far as to perform mastectomies prophylactically on high-risk patients. In Britain, while mastectomy, in one form or another has been the routine treatment, as yet surgeons are not known to have recommended high-risk patients to have their breasts removed to stop them from developing breast cancer.

The changes in the law on informed consent in some states of the USA has been backed by information provided by the federal government that helps the patient to ask the right questions. You need to know what the questions are in order to ask them. All too frequently a doctor says to a patient, 'Have you any questions?' and the patient, ignorant as most of us are about medical practices and the workings of our bodies, tamely answers, 'No.' The leaflet published by the US Department of Health and Human Services, called *What You Need to Know about Cancer of the Breast*, goes some way towards providing basic information, so that a woman may ask the right questions. However, the framework of reference is entirely that of orthodox medicine. The leaflet is informational, briefly describing breast cancer, forms of diagnosis and forms of treatment. For further information it lists telephone numbers in each state which you can call 'toll free' to get a Cancer Information Service. Research is discussed as well as rehabilitation, and a glossary is included explaining relevant medical words. All this is brief but makes a good, useful, informational starting-point for a woman who may have breast cancer. It goes much further than similar leaflets published in this country which deal mainly with how you examine your own breasts. Southampton is one of the few authorities to provide the kind of useful information needed by a patient through its organization called Help for Health Service.

They issue a handbook on breast cancer which gives information, a reading list of useful books and addresses of relevant organizations. It is the kind of information that all local authorities should provide or, as in the USA, the relevant government department, the Department of Health and Social Security (DHSS), should make sure it is provided by publishing it themselves.

The most interesting part of the USA leaflet is the section entitled 'Questions You May Want to Ask Your Doctor'. This is followed by a list of questions it recommends that patients ask. Unaccustomed to being encouraged to ask questions, this list would come to the NHS patient as a shock, particularly in the case of some of the questions it suggests.

Questions you may want to ask your doctor
You or your family may find it difficult to ask your doctor some of the questions you may have. This is understandable. Cancer and its treatment are complex. Even your doctor may not always be able to give definite answers. But he or she should discuss your questions with you. Some typical questions might include these:
- Is the tumour benign or malignant?
- If it is cancer, what kind do I have?
- If it is cancer, has it spread?
- Can you predict how sucessful an operation or other treatment would be?
- What are the risks?
- Should I get an opinion from another doctor?
- If an operation is done will I need further treatment?
- What about the possibility of breast reconstruction?
- Is it possible to resume normal activities afterwards?
- If I take anti-cancer drugs, what will the side effects be?
- How often will I need medical check-ups?
- What should I tell my friends and relatives?

We have used this list as our starting-point, adding to it additional questions that we think important to ask.

Obviously not everyone needs to ask all these questions. If the answer to the first is that the tumour is not cancerous (benign), then the questions will be different from those to be asked if it is cancerous (malignant). We have not confined ourselves to orthodox medicine. Questions must also be asked of alternative and complementary medicine. Armed with these questions and the reasons why they should be asked, we hope that a woman with a breast disorder will be better equipped to give informed consent to any form of treatment.

Michael Baum, Professor of Surgery at King's College Hospital, in his book *Breast Cancer: The Facts* argues, 'women should trust the medical profession that they are working for the benefit of womankind, once this trust is lost there is no hope at all.' Doctors have to *earn* trust – or rather they have now to *win* back the trust that we innocently had in them and that they have, in differing degrees, lost. Trust is a two-way relationship based on mutual respect. Better-informed patients can no longer be treated in the paternalistic and autocratic manner of the past. Doctors who trust and respect their patients are much more likely to be respected and trusted in turn. In the words of Jory Graham, an American who has battled for many years with cancer:

> As a doctrine and as a practical reality, informed consent is neither so complicated nor so difficult as doctors and lawyers would make it, nor is there any good reason for the medical debates it engenders. At its core, it is respect for the patient as an individual, not a defense against the possibility of a later malpractice suit.

Women have changed the way doctors treat them in pregnancy and childbirth. The changes they have made in maternity services mark one of the major consumer victories of the last decade or two. Pregnancy and childbirth has become a more humane experience. Those who have lobbied for change can claim significant improvements. Such change is possible in other areas of medicine. Medicine can be humanized, but the process of humanization will inevitably be spearheaded by those whom it most concerns: that is the patients. Alternative medicine offers a human approach and orthodox medicine, even if it refuses to learn anything from alternative medicine, could learn from its attitude to patients.

Asking questions is a central part of establishing with your doctor or surgeon that you are a person and not just a body to be treated. The first question any woman attending a breast clinic will ask and will want answered honestly is 'Is my lump cancerous or non-cancerous?' For over 80 per cent of these women with a lump and/or other symptoms the answer will be that she does not have cancer. If the woman is under 30 the chances that her lump is cancerous are very, very slight. It is over the age of 35 that the incidence of breast cancer really starts to rise.

Our society regards the word cancer as a taboo word and its usage is still evaded, particularly by doctors in talking to their patients. Surgeons often either use medical terminology, frequently not understood by the patient, or use terms like 'nasty', 'bad news' or 'it doesn't look good'. It is often the patient herself who wants and needs the word spelt out clearly to grasp the reality. Breaking the news to a woman that she has breast cancer is not an easy task, but there are many more sensitive ways of doing it than by putting an 'x' on the affected breast or telling her quite baldly that she has cancer and, in the next sentence, informing her when the breast can be cut off.

For the majority whose lumps and other symptoms are not cancerous (benign) there are also questions to be asked. In the euphoria of relief it is hard to collect one's thoughts and ask the relevant questions. It is even harder if you have just been told that you have breast cancer to recover enough from the traumatic news to ask anything at all. The surgeon will almost certainly suggest to you, immediately after telling you that you have cancer, what treatment he or she thinks you should have. It is crucial, unless you are absolutely sure that the treatment suggested corresponds with what you want, to ask for time. Ask for time to think, for time to be able to ask questions and discuss alternatives, and time to be sure that the decision you are making is the right one for you. Some doctors feel that both patient and doctor should pause for thought at this crucial moment, enabling both doctor and patient to consider the alternatives. With the exception of the few fast-growing breast cancers, and they are the exception, a few days or even a week or two will not make the difference between life and death. It may well, however, make the difference between being able to confront your own disease or not. Remember you are the one who has to live with your body.

7. Breast cancer

The consultant then said, 'I do think it's cancer'. No he didn't, he said, 'It's something nasty', and I said, 'Do you mean cancer? and he said, 'Yes.'

(Jenny)

I was sitting on my bed at five to seven and I heard the curtains woosh and as I looked up there was the registrar and the houseman standing there at the end of the bed saying, 'Mrs X, I'm afraid we've got bad news for you. Your biopsy proved malignant.'

(Hazel)

Cancer of the breast: what is it?

Cancer of the breast is in one sense no different from cancer in any other part of the body. Its central feature is the uncontrolled reproduction of cells. Our bodies are constructed of billions of cells, each one having a particular function. When the body is working normally, each cell is kept under control doing its allotted job. If a cell starts reproducing in an uncontrolled fashion then, except when it happens in the blood-forming cells, it causes a growth or swelling. Not all growths are cancerous. The difference between cancerous (malignant) and non-cancerous (benign) growths is that in the latter, although the cells divide quickly, they remain under control. The growth that such doubling causes remains contained, neither invading surrounding tissue, nor spreading to other parts of the body. Except when such growths occur in places like the brain or the liver, where they can cause fatal obstructions, they are rarely serious. A fibroadenoma (see section on non-cancerous breast disorders) is an example of this type of non-cancerous growth that happens quite frequently in the breast.

In contrast to benign growths cancerous growths invade surrounding tissue and can spread. This happens when some of the cancerous cells, often referred to as 'rogue cells', break away and, as it were, 'swim off' to settle like a time-bomb somewhere else in the body. The cancerous growth from which the rogue cells break away is called the primary tumour, and 'secondaries' are formed when rogue cells start off the process of uncontrolled proliferation somewhere else in the body. This spread to another part of the body is called 'metastasis'. Unfortunately cancer cells do not just divide too quickly but in the process of doing so they lose their ability to perform their specialist functions. So instead of being useful, as cells should be, keeping the body ticking over in good working order, they become useless. Not only do they become useless but they also become greedy parasites invading other areas of the body, not just as part of their growth but in order to seek nutrition. This process happens at the expense of normal healthy tissue. Cancerous cells are like a growing, invading, hungry army which has, as part of its force, a long-range strike potential.

If it is cancer, what kind do I have?

Some women feel cancer is cancer – 'Do I need to know more?' Knowing more is important. It helps to understand what is wrong, and where, and to guide both the surgeon and you in making a decision about treatment. For those women whose cancer is confirmed while they are unconscious and who have agreed before the anaesthetic that the surgeon may perform whatever surgery he or she thinks necessary cannot ask this question in relation to their primary treatment. This form of instant surgical treatment not only denies the woman a chance to discuss her treatment but also means that the surgeon is acting on the limited information got from the analysis of a frozen section which can only confirm, or otherwise, the presence of cancerous cells. Further detailed information cannot be gathered in the brief time that this analysis takes. It is hoped that changed attitudes and changed methods will make the 'frozen section' a thing of the past. Meanwhile it is important for those women still having frozen sections to know what kind of cancer they have, for while the decision about primary treatment is taken instantly, that knowledge is important to discussions about any further treatment thought necessary.

Cancers are named by the parts of the body in which they occur and by the type of tissue in which the original, primary growth is found. Breast cancer almost always originates in the breast, which is why it is called 'breast cancer'. It is very rare for a rogue cell from a cancerous growth in another part of the body to find its way to the breast and cause a secondary growth there. The type of tissue in which the growth occurs determines whether the cancer is called a 'carcinoma' or a 'sarcoma'. Carcinoma is the name used to describe cancers that occur in the cells that line ducts in different parts of the body. In the breast, carcinomas occur in the cells lining the ducts and lobules of the milk production system (see Diagram 1). Cancers that grow in muscles, fat, bone, etc. (the connective tissues) are called sarcomas and they can also occur, although fairly rarely, in the breasts.

Once cancer is identified, further analysis can tell more about its kind. This analysis is done in the pathology laboratory and so if your surgeon says, 'We are waiting for the path report', or reads your 'path' report, this kind of further detail should be contained in it. Common to all cancers is the uncontrolled duplication of cells, but each individual cancer has its own way of behaving. Further analysis can help to predict the possible ways in which it will behave and thus help in the decision whether one form of treatment or another will be beneficial. At one end of the range there are cancerous cells which keep some of the characteristics of the original cell from which they grew. At the other are cells which look nothing like their original forms. The cancer is graded for its malignancy according to the

Diagram I THE BREAST INSIDE

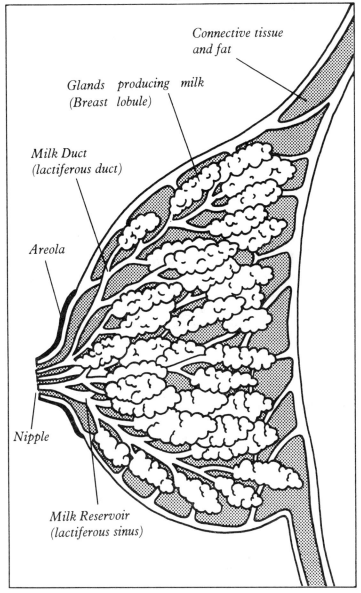

Connective tissue
and fat

Glands producing milk
(Breast lobule)

Milk Duct
(lactiferous duct)

Areola

Nipple

Milk Reservoir
(lactiferous sinus)

place of the cancer cells in this range. Those most like their parent cells are the least potentially harmful or, put another way, the ones which give the best long-term outlook. However, this information can only indicate the way a cancer is likely to behave; cancer is highly unpredictable and the rule is only proved by its many, many exceptions.

It is also important to know whether your cancer is hormone dependent or independent. This knowledge can be a deciding factor in opting for certain forms of treatment rather than others. It has long been known that breast cancer is linked to hormonal activity, although the exact links are not clear. In the past surgeons found that if they removed a woman's ovaries (oopherectomy) then recurrence or spread of breast cancer could be lessened or controlled for a time. The operation was often performed routinely, and still is by some surgeons, following a mastectomy regardless of whether the cancer was of a kind that would respond to such treatment. It is now possible to determine whether a breast cancer is dependent or inde-pendent of the hormone oestrogen by doing a test which is called an ER assay (an oestrogen receptor test). If the results of this show the cancer to be oestrogen dependent then it will probably respond to hormone treatment, but if independent then other forms of treatment would probably be more effective. This information is particularly useful in a case of recurrence. If it has been gathered from the first biopsy, it can be kept and acted upon immediately cancer recurs.

All the information about the kind of cancer you have is contained in the biopsy report, which is not shown to you. It is part of the 'secret' records kept by the hospital about you. It seems a perfectly reasonable request to make that you be allowed to see your biopsy report, if only to see and check the evidence for yourself. One woman, years after a mastectomy, still harboured a lingering doubt expressed in the words, 'I never saw the biopsy report. Perhaps . . .' If reading the biopsy report dispels doubts, ask to see it and, if you don't understand the code language, ask to have it explained.

How far has it gone and has it spread?

Besides knowing what kind of cancer you have, it is crucial to know how far it has spread locally within the breast and whether it has spread to other parts of the body. This information should have a direct bearing on what form of treatment would be most effective.

Doctors commonly decide how far the cancer has spread by looking at three key factors – the size of the original tumour, whether and how much the lymph nodes are involved (see below for an explanation), and whether it has spread (distant metastasis) to other parts of the body. With that information they 'stage' the cancer. The staging system provides the basis for decisions about treatment and gives an indication of the patient's outlook. The system stages breast cancer between I and IV, stage I patients having a good chance of a cure and stage IV patients having a very poor outlook.

Stage I : the cancerous tumour in the breast is less than five centimetres in diameter and there is no evidence of lymph node involvement or distant spread.
Stage II : the tumour in the breast is no bigger than five centimetres with some lymph node involvement but no distant spread.
Stage III : The primary tumour is bigger than five centimetres; there is evidence of local advancement such as peau d'orange (that is, when the skin surface looks like orange peel); ulceration of the skin; fixation and the lymph nodes are involved.
Stage IV : there is evidence of spread to other parts of the body as well as local advancement (spread) and lymph node involvement.

Many doctors now believe that pathological staging based on whether the cancer is poorly or well differentiated (see previous section for explanation) provides a much better guide to the outlook. Lymph node involvement has always been central to

39

the outlook of a patient: as a rule of thumb, the more extensive the lymph node involvement the poorer the outlook for the patient. However, although the extent of lymph node involvement remains an important element in the staging of breast cancer it is only one element and one which is subject to some questioning because of the imprecise knowledge of the exact functioning of the lymph nodes.

Lymph nodes are to be found all over the body, but those important to breast cancer are to be found in the underarm area. That is why doctors examining you for breast cancer always feel under the arm for any swelling. Lymph nodes are small masses of gland tissue through which lymph, a colourless fluid, drains and is purified. They are part of the body's vital defence against disease. As such they can act both as a blocker to cancerous cells travelling from the breast to other parts of the body or as a conductor of them. They act as a blocker in that the lymph nodes contain things called lymphocytes and histiocytes which are fighters against cancerous cells. However, as a draining system, like the blood stream, the lymph nodes provide a channel though which cancerous cells can pass. Swelling in the underarm area does not always mean adverse lymph node involvement. It may just be that the nodes are swollen from extra activity fighting the cancerous cells.

This dual function of the lymph nodes has led to questioning both of the staging syste and the conventional ways of treating breast cancer based on it. Some believe that if the lymph nodes are involved then cancer will already have spread to other parts of the body and therefore treatment should not just be local, that is, to the breast area, but should be to the body as a whole. If the lymph nodes were involved they were often surgically removed or killed by radiotherapy. This too has been questioned on the basis that removing all the lymph nodes is removing part of the body's potential fighting force.

Finally the staging system has also been questioned, because it does not take into consideration whether the cancer is oestrogen dependent or independent. Hormone treatment is now changing the outlook positively for women even with breast cancer which has spread to other parts of the body. Perhaps nowadays the greatest use of the staging system is that it provides a means by which doctors can assess whether progress is being made in the treatment of breast cancer. By comparing patients with similar staged breast cancer and measuring whether those treated recently are doing better than those in the past, some assessment can be made as to whether new forms of treatment or combinations of treatment are giving women a better outlook.

One curiosity about the staging system, and indeed about decisions made about treatment of breast cancer is that they are made in relation to whether there is distant spread, metastasis, but often they do not have the evidence on which to make the judgement. Most women undergo surgery for breast cancer without having had a bone and liver scan to find out if it has spread to either, these being the places breast cancer is most likely to spread to. Many women may well feel they would like to know if the cancer is more likely to spread before deciding on surgery. A bone and liver scan are two ways of finding out about how far or if it has spread. One of the more disturbing stories recounted about breast cancer was of a woman who died of cancer six weeks after having had a mastectomy. Had tests been done she may well have chosen not to have undergone the trauma of surgery. If cancer is diagnosed then before deciding on any form of treatment it would be wise to ask to have a bone and liver scan.

A liver scan is done by injecting a radioactive substance into the bloodstream which is absorbed by the liver blood supply and is then scanned with a gamma camera. It takes relatively little time and is painless, although this test, like the bone scan, involves the use of a radioactive substance and radioactivity has its risks. A bone scan works on the same basis; a radioactive substance is injected which is absorbed by the bone structure. This process takes longer as there is a wait while the 'dye' filters around the body and the scanning process can also take an hour or more.

Having been looked at, felt, scanned and with the evidence of

41

a full biopsy report, you and the surgeon have an array of information on which to start discussions about the form of treatment you the patient might choose. There is one further vital question to ask which may affect the discussion and that is whether you are in a trial area.

Is this a trial area?

Clinical trials are carried out in all areas of medicine. As a consequence of the outrage at the end of the Second World War when it was revealed that the Nazis had used prisoners as human guinea pigs for a variety of medical experiments, the Nuremberg Code was drawn up. This laid down certain rules of conduct for doctors and scientists involved in human experimentation. The basis of the Nuremberg Code and all its successors is that of informed consent – that is, that a patient, having been *fully* informed of a trial, its nature, duration, hazards and objectives, should then be free, without any pressure, to choose voluntarily whether to take part. Sadly this does not always happen. Sometimes patients are never informed or find out after the event that they were participants in a trial and that the treatment they were given was 'chosen for them' not even by a doctor but by a computer.

The question of trials is an important one to breast disorders and breast cancer in particular. There have been and still are several trials conducted in the search for more effective treatment. Trials have been conducted in the treatment of breast cancer on the use of different types of surgery and on different combinations of treatment, for example, lumpectomy (removal of the lump) versus mastectomy, and surgery plus radiotherapy versus surgery alone. These trials have arisen because doctors are deeply divided about the treatment of breast cancer and until a treatment is found that clearly achieves better results, trials are likely to be conducted.

Before agreeing to any treatment you should ask if you are in a trial area and whether your treatment is part of a trial. If so then you should be informed of all aspects of the trial and it should be made quite clear that you need only participate in it if you want to.

Trial methods vary. In breast cancer they are often based on giving two sets of women with similar symptoms different treatments and then following up the cases to see if there is any significant difference in recurrence, cure and survival rates.

In the testing of anti-cancer drugs, randomized controlled clinical trials are often used. This means that an anti-cancer drug is tested against a control group not taking that particular drug. In this form of trial it is neither the doctor nor the patient who decides which drug (or placebo) will be prescribed, but the computer at the trial centre from which the trial is administered. It is an extremely questionable form of testing drugs. As a form of testing it may be 'scientific', but scientific precision often fails to recognize the individuality of human beings, their bodies, their particular manifestation of a disease and their relationship with a doctor.

If you do consent to take part in a trial, you should also be fully aware that it is your right to withdraw from the trial at any point if for some reason you wish to do so. You should only agree to take part in a trial when you have been fully informed about its nature, have given your written consent and have also been made aware of your right to withdraw from it. Of doctors who do not inform or explain to their patients that they are part of a trial, Carolyn Faulder in *Whose Body Is It?* writes:

> Personally I find it hard to understand how any doctor can live with his conscience knowing that he has put patients into a breast cancer trial or any similar study in which patients are likely to have strong preferences or indeed a completely different order of priorities from his own, without *giving* them the opportunity to decide whether they are prepared to accept a randomized allocation of treatments. Truly, this is playing God with a vengeance.

Can you predict how successful an operation or other treatment would be?

Doctors don't like predicting, yet they have been known to tell women that unless they accept a particular form of treatment then their life will be shortened. This kind of 'threatening' prediction is bullying of the worst sort and has been used on women refusing a mastectomy. Most doctors are wary of predicting and rightly so, for breast cancer behaves unpredictably. Michael Baum in his book *Breast Cancer* writes:

> Finally, we also recognize that the disease does not behave as a single entity but has an extraordinarily wide biological variation in behaviour, with some women dying of the disease with an almost undetectable primary tumour, whereas others may live for many years having refused treatment in the first place.

He then cites two cases to illustrate this extreme variability. Case one was a woman who had barely detectable cancerous cells in her breast and died 18 months after diagnosis. The other was of a woman aged 60 who refused the advice of her doctor that her cancerous tumour be treated by a radical mastectomy. Thirty years later, aged 90, she once again attended the clinic, having outlived the doctor and three husbands. The original tumour had slowly grown over the 30 years and another had developed in her other breast, but there was no evidence of spread to other parts of her body. Of this case Michael Baum comments, 'It is unlikely that radical mastectomy 30 years ago would have improved on this outcome.' The best a doctor can do is to advise on which form of treatment or combination of treatments would give the best outlook.

Which treatment – surgery, radiotherapy, chemotherapy or hormone treatment?

As we have said before, combinations of treatment are often used in the treatment of breast cancer. The development of 'adjuvant therapy', the use of additional treatment to surgery, arose from the realization that surgery alone often failed to stop either local or distant spread of the cancer. It also failed to treat the distant spread (metastasis) that has already happened in some cases by the time of the operation. In brief, additional (adjuvant) therapy was developed because surgery alone proved to be, in many cases, a not very successful form of treating breast cancer. As breast cancer surgery has become more conservative, more sophisticated forms of radiotherapy, chemotherapy and hormone therapy have been developed. While these additional therapies are usually used as a safety measure following surgery, sometimes they are used on their own as a primary treatment. It is because of the bad track record of surgery alone and the increasingly effective use of the other forms of treatment that discussion about treatment should consider all possibilities. Each form of treatment has both its benefits and its risks, its after-effects and its side-effects, all of which should be known.

Surgery
The primary and often the only form of treatment for breast cancer for most of this century has been surgery. Indeed until recently other forms of treatment were not even considered. In the past the question was, and mostly still is, not whether surgery should be performed but how extensive it should be.

Debate has raged recently and continues to rage over the use of different kinds of surgery and their effectiveness. One question that is rarely raised is whether surgery should be used at all. It has not been one of the medical success stories of this century. The mortality figures from breast cancer have not decreased since the Second World War, although there is now hope that the corner might have been turned. One doubt that hangs over the use of surgery and which has never satisfactorily been dispelled since there has been little research into it is whether surgery itself can aid the spread of cancerous cells, particularly their distant spread. This is hotly denied by most surgeons who claim that there is no evidence to support the suspicion. However, to a lay person it is hard to understand why

45

surgical intervention cannot lead to some disturbed rogue cells slipping into the bloodstream at the time of surgery. The fact that surgeons often suggest a course of chemotherapy following surgery to 'mop up' any shedding of cancerous cells caused by surgery confirms the suspicion, as does the fact that local cancers occasionally recur at the original site of surgery.

But for most doctors and lay people alike, cutting the cancer out seems the obvious form of treatment. The debate over surgery has therefore not been whether or not to use it but over what kind. In most British hospitals breast cancer is still 'treated' by some form of mastectomy. This is despite the fact that recent trials have shown that in patients with similar stages of breast cancer there is *no* appreciable difference in the long-term survival rates between those treated with different types of surgery and those on whom mastectomies were performed. In the light of such evidence more and more patients and some surgeons are questioning the almost routine use of mastectomy.

This questioning has led to an increase in the range of surgery used in the treatment of breast cancer. The decision is based on the amount of breast tissue, surrounding tissue and muscle that is to be removed. At one end is the removal of the lump only (a lumpectomy) and at the other is the 'extended or super-radical mastectomy', now rarely performed, which removes the breast, the surrounding muscles and the underarm area (see Diagram 2). Between these two, one kind can blur into another – a large lumpectomy can be almost like having a simple mastectomy, etc. The general trend over the last few years has been towards the removal of less of the surrounding tissue and muscles. Some surgeons are increasingly trying to preserve the breast itself, especially in cases where there is little local spread and no lymph node involvement.

In considering what form of surgery, many factors have to be weighed. Women vary greatly in their feelings about having a breast removed. Whatever those feelings, they are important and should be considered. The after-effects of surgery should also be taken into account. A mastectomy is not just cosmetically mutilating, causing women deep emotional trauma, it can,

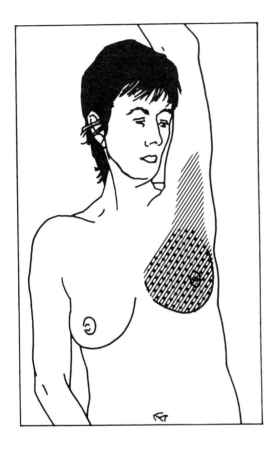

Diagram II

*Area removed
by an extended
mastectomy.*

*Area removed
by a simple
mastectomy.*

depending on the kind of mastectomy, cause a variety of physical after-effects. If some or all of the surrounding muscles are removed, the use of the body can be affected; the more muscles removed, the greater the effect. Exercises and physiotherapy can help to get back some of the usage but not all. The removal of the lymph nodes can cause problems of swelling in the operated arm. This swelling is called lymphoedema and is caused by the fluid, normally drained by the lymphatic drainage system, being unable to drain away. The swelling can be disfiguring, uncomfortable and even painful. The physical after-effects are

47

therefore almost in direct proportion to the extensiveness of the surgery. Other physical effects are dependent on the size and shape of the woman herself. A woman with very small breasts will suffer less problem of weight imbalance, of feeling lopsided, and therefore have less problem in adjusting to renewed weight distribution. For women with large breasts this can present quite a problem.

In discussing surgery it is important to clarify exactly what the surgeon intends removing and why. This should be part of the general discussion with the surgeon about treatment. It becomes of particular importance, indeed crucial importance, when you, as a patient, are presented with a consent form to sign. A consent form must be signed by the patient before any surgery can take place. Since what you sign to on the consent form is of such importance, we reproduce here a typical one. It is a copy of the one used by the Central Middlesex Hospital and is standard. We have omitted only the additional line for a parent or guardian to sign in the case of a child.

First, it should be noted that on the consent form the operation to be undergone is specified and also specified is the obligation of the medical practitioner to explain 'the nature and purpose of the operation' – but not its risks or side-effects. While the patient signs for a particular operation she is also expected to sign a *carte blanche* for the surgeon to take 'such further or alternative operative measures as maybe found necessary during the course of the above mentioned (specified) operation'. This means that once you have signed this form any part of your body can be operated on while you are on the operating table. You may go to sleep thinking that you will wake up having had a lump removed but you could find that your appendix, ovaries, breast and big toe have gone and you would have signed away your legal right to complain. This may be a ludicrous and unlikely example, but it is not uncommon to find women who have consented to one form of surgery discovering when they wake up that much more extensive surgery than they expected had been performed.

The form says that 'deletions, insertions or amendments to

CONSENT FOR OPERATION

I .... of ....
.... hereby consent

to undergo the operation of ....
the nature and purpose of which have been

explained to me by Dr/Mr ....
I also consent to such further or alternative
operative measures as may be found necessary
during the course of the above mentioned
operation and to the administration of general,
local or other anaesthetics for any of these
purposes. No assurance has been given to me that
the operation will be performed by any particular
practitioner.

Date .... Signed ....
(Patient)
I confirm that I have explained the nature and
purpose of this operation to the patient.

Date .... Signed ....
(Medical Practitioner)

*Any deletions, insertions or amendments to the
form are to be made before the explanation is
given and the form submitted for signature.*

---

the form are to be made before the explanation is given and the form submitted for signature'. This is clearly directed at the medical practitioner and not at the patient. Nowhere on the form does it say that the patient has the right to delete, insert or amend anything, yet they may and it is their right to do so. Most patients want to delete the sentence consenting to any 'further or alternative operative measures' and by doing so signalling

49

consent only to the specified operation. In the case of breast surgery this might mean consent only to a lumpectomy. The surgeon then cannot, on 'opening the patient up', there and then make the decision to proceed to more extensive surgery. Some women are happy to agree to the removal of anything the surgeon thinks fit. Others would prefer to take their disease in stages, having time to think and to discuss it at each stage. If it is the latter course you wish to pursue, then be sure to amend the consent form making your wishes quite clear before signing it.

Again, while some patients may not mind who performs their surgery others may feel strongly that they wish a particular surgeon to do so. If you feel strongly then the section which states that 'No assurance has been given to me that the operation will be performed by any particular practitioner' should be accordingly amended. In NHS hospitals it is difficult to get the form amended to stipulate a particular surgeon but if you have confidence in a particular person then you should try to get a written assurance that that person will perform the operation.

It is well worth studying this consent form calmly and away from the hospital in order to be equipped to deal with it when presented to you. This often happens when you are stressed, alone in hospital and very frequently under sedation, since hospitals have a habit of bringing the form round for signing on the evening prior to the operation. If you have not got a friend, husband or relative with you when asked to sign it, take a deep breath, read it carefully and if you are not happy with what you are required to sign insist that it is changed until you are. This is often much easier if you have someone with you. Alone or supported, remember it is your body, your life and *you* have the final word about it.

Breast reconstruction Breast reconstruction has been hailed by some as the great breakthrough for women with breast cancer, giving them new hope with a new breast. An article in the *Guardian* of 18 July 1985 entitled 'Where the Woman Comes First' opened with the following paragraph: 'Betty Graham was shocked to find she had breast cancer in June 1983, thoroughly apprehensive at the thought of a mastectomy and euphoric the morning after the operation. There, where there ought to have been two breasts . . . were two breasts.' Unquestioningly this was accepted as a step forward echoing the sentiments expressed in Carolyn Faulder's book *Breast Cancer*, in which she devotes a whole chapter to silicone implants and breast reconstructions calling it 'A New Hope'.

A real new hope for women would be a cure and a more hopeful future would be the treatment of breast cancer that does not involve radical surgery. Breast reconstruction offers neither of those hopes and in itself poses many problems. Our discussion of it here under the general heading 'Surgery' is not only because in itself it involves surgery, but primary surgery (mastectomy) is increasingly offered with a sweetener – 'Oh well, you can have an implant or reconstruction.' Women thus agree to the removal of their breast because it can be replaced or reconstructed. It is totally understandable that women faced with the loss of a breast should find that bitter pill easier to swallow if the breast can be replaced – even if artificially. For those who have had successful implants or reconstruction done, it does provide a way of coping with mutilation and being able to live with their body. For them it has made life following a mastectomy more bearable.

Breast reconstruction, however, reverses the trend in the treatment of breast cancer. It leads to more surgery not less. It is usually done following a mastectomy and therefore perpetuates the use of mastectomies when that form of surgery is increasingly being questioned. The general surgical trend is towards more conservative surgery, with more and more women being treated by the removal of the lump only usually followed by other treatment.

Besides questioning breast reconstruction because it is based on an acceptance of radical surgery, it is also questionable because the process itself is hazardous. A few women, like Betty Graham, have an implant placed at the time of initial surgery. Many surgeons do not offer such treatment and for many women it is not possible to have an implant at the time of surgery. Women who have radiotherapy following surgery cannot have an implant until the course of radiotherapy is finished. But they can undergo the process of tissue expansion which aids the subsequent insertion of an implant. Tissue expansion means re-opening the mastectomy scar tissue by two inches or so and inserting a round bag with a tube attachment. The bag is inflated with a saline solution, the quantity being increased over a period of weeks causing the tissue to expand. When it has expanded enough the bag is removed and a silicone implant inserted. The incision is then restitched causing no secondary scars.

Many women told at the time of their mastectomies that they could, if they so wished, return for reconstructive surgery later do not do so. A year or two later they have learned to live with their bodies and find the idea of further surgical intervention distasteful.

Silicone gel implants are in themselves questionable. There are those who believe that they are potentially carcinogenic, that is, that they may cause cancer. This has not been proved but it is a worry that some doctors have expressed about the use of it in breast reconstruction. Whilst the procedure of 'popping in' a silicone implant sounds simple in practice, it is often difficult and by no means always produces the desired effect, either cosmetically or medically. The body can reject the silicone implant just as it can other foreign bodies. This can be painful, distressing and lead to further surgery. One of the dangers of using a silicone implant following surgery for breast cancer is that the implant can conceal any future local recurrence of cancer in the breast. Finally implants don't change with ageing. The artificially created symmetrical breasts can, with time, become asymmetrical.

There is no question that for some women, breast reconstruction is physically and psychologically successful, but for many more it is not. It certainly should not be seen as 'the new hope' and if you are considering it it is worth considering first whether a mastectomy is really necessary and whether more conservative surgery in the first place would be a better option. It is not surprising that in the USA where surgeons make big money out of surgery that they are enthusiastically offering women the additional surgery of silicone implants. While increasing numbers of British surgeons claim to be more sensitive now to the emotional trauma of losing a breast, one would hope that sensitivity would lead them actively to search for treatments that conserve the breast not replace it.

Radiotherapy
Radiotherapy is a means of treating the disease by using radiation energy. Surgery is used to cut the cancer out. Radiation, the basis of radiotherapy, is used to burn it out. Radiotherapy has been used for a long time now in the treatment of breast cancer. It is mainly used following surgery as a means of trying to ensure that any cancerous cells left in and around the breast area after surgery are mopped up. Sometimes, though rarely, it is used as a form of primary treament. It is also used to treat local recurrence and to alleviate pain in cases of advanced cancer.

Radiotherapy is usually given with high energy X-ray beams to an area that has been carefully selected. The course of radiotherapy, its length, the dosage and the area to be treated is decided by a radiotherapist. The treatment suggested will be based on the size and shape of the tumour, whether it is fast or slow growing and whether the cancer is well or poorly differentiated. Other factors will also be considered, like the age and state of health of the patient and other treatments undergone or proposed. A radiographer is the person who actually administers the treatment.

The course of treatment involves attending the hospital as an out-patient everyday, except for weekends, usually for about ten weeks. At the first visit your skin will be marked with lines detailing the exact area to be treated. You are asked not to wash the marks off and, indeed not to wash the treated area during the course of treatment at all. Each session lasts for about half an hour, although that can vary enormously according to 'waiting time', the actual X-ray not taking long.

A course of radiotherapy while not painful is, or can be, distressing and uncomfortable. It is distressing since regular attendance at the hospital is a daily reminder of the cancer. The radiotherapy itself can have various immediate side-effects. For example, it can cause a skin reaction like sunburn particularly with fair skins. The ban on washing the area can cause it to itch. This is often worse for women with large breasts who get chafing under the breast where it rubs the chest wall and for women whose course of treatment takes place in hot weather. The other main side-effects are nausea, fatigue and depression. Like the other side-effects these vary in degree for different patients, some barely suffering from any while others may find them almost incapacitating. Whatever the degree these side-effects come to an end with the end of the treatment.

Radiotherapy can cause long term-damage. The most common kind is the development of bands of fibrous tissue which can restrict mobility in the upper arm and shoulder. This can be accentuated by the drying up of the lubrication in the treated muscles, thus reducing their elasticity, mobility and effectiveness. Lymph glands can also be damaged, which leads to an increase in the swelling of the treated arm. While these long-term effects are not uncommon, radiotherapy carefully controlled and administered by skilled hands should mean that they are reduced to a minimum.

Apart from the known short-term and long-term side-effects of radiotherapy there is considerable debate about other possible long-term side-effects. Brenda Kidman in her book *A Gentle Way With Cancer* describes how she, like so many other women, had radiotherapy following surgery for breast cancer to 'mop up' any cancer cells that had been left behind. Of her treatment she wrote:

In three weeks I was given 3,500 rems. The recommended maximum safety level for those working in X-ray departments is five rems over a period of one year. But as it was pointed out when I requested to know the exact amount of radiation exposure given to me, cancer patients are special cases. The same safety regulations do not apply and consultants are entitled to take 'justifiable risks' on behalf of the cancer patient without explaining what these risks entail.

Brenda Kidman's concern about the often routine use of radiotherapy as a mopping up treatment is justifiable and shared by some orthodox practitioners.

There have been several trials in different countries to test whether radiotherapy achieves better and longer-term control of the disease. The results have been contradictory, with different trials using different doses of radiation and looking for different things, some measuring local recurrence and some measuring long-term survival prospects. It has been found in some trials that radiotherapy does reduce the local recurrence rate, but others have shown that it has not led to any increase in the long-term survival rate. Claims have been made, and also challenged, that women who have had radiotherapy have an increased chance of developing distant spread of the disease in the bone, lung, liver and skin. There are those that argue that the routine use of post-operative radiotherapy in the treatment of breast cancer should be made obsolete. Such use exposes a majority of women to radiation unnecessarily to protect the 20 or 30 per cent of women who do develop local recurrence. Radiotherapy should, they argue, be used on those 20 or 30 per cent as and when local recurrence occurs. There are those who oppose the use of radiotherapy altogether, arguing that it does more long-term harm than short term good. Dr Jan Stjernesward of the Swiss Institute for Experimental Cancer Research has argued that 'Stopping the routine use of prophylactic, local radiotherapy could increase survival rates.' He claimed women who had surgery alone did better than women who had been irradiated. This claim has also been made following trials in the USA, where women who were not irradiated did better in terms of long-term survival than those who were.

As more surgeons conserve more of the breast the old method of treating cancerous tumours internally is being revived. In the

1930s attempts were made to treat breast cancer with radium needles. Recent treatment has the same principle behind it but uses radioactive irridium wires threaded through the tumour. For this the patient has to go into hospital for a few days to have the wires inserted, to stay while they are treating her and then to have the wires removed before returning home. This treatment does not cause the damage to the muscles that X-ray treatment can but it uses very high doses of radiation in the area treated. Such high doses must be a cause for concern.

As yet no trial has conclusively proved whether or not radiotherapy affects the long-term survival rates of breast cancer patients. For a lay person, that the treating of cancer with radiation, something that is known to cause cancer, can also cure it is something of a mystery. There is no doubt, however, that radiation on differentiated cancer cells does cause them to shrink. The doubt must remain for the time being on the long-term effects. It is clearly an area where more research is needed. Meanwhile women should question the routine use of radiotherapy following surgery. Nowadays it is often used as 'one treatment', a lumpectomy followed by radiotherapy being offered as opposed to mastectomy. As with any treatment, you should choose which of the options or the risks you would rather take.

Chemotherapy

Surgery is designed to cut the cancer out, radiotherapy to burn it out and chemotherapy to poison it. Surgery and radiotherapy are aimed at getting the disease under control locally; this means making sure that all the cancerous cells in the breast and in the area immediately around the breast including the lymph nodes are cut out and killed off. Chemotherapy is aimed at poisoning any cancerous cells that may have been carried off through the bloodstream or the lymphatic channels to distant parts of the body, though research into the use of chemotherapy for the primary tumour itself is now being done.

Chemotherapy is the use of cytotoxic drugs. These are chemicals which damage growing cells. To date no drug has been developed that attacks cancerous cells only leaving the healthy ones undamaged. Cytotoxic drugs which can and do destroy fast-growing cells are used, but they also destroy or damage healthy fast-growing cells as well as those which are cancerous. Since their first use in the 1940s, better cytotoxic drugs have been developed – better in the sense that they are more specific, damaging fewer healthy cells and causing less severe side-effects, even though they still act on the body as a whole and not just on the cancerous cells.

At first, cytotoxic drugs were only used in the treatment of breast cancer in its advanced stages. The treatment was designed not to achieve a cure but to try to control the cancer and give the patient some remission from the disease. The disadvantage of its use at this stage, when high dosages are given, is that the side-effects caused by the toxic (poisonous) drugs can be a very high price to pay for an extended life. These drugs are still used to try to control the disease in its advanced stages, but they are also now sometimes used as part of the 'primary package' of treatment. Almost all patients given this dosage of cytotoxic drugs suffered one or more of the following side-effects – loss of hair, vomiting/nausea, constipation/diarrhoea, numbness in the fingertips, mouth ulceration, abdominal pain and a general state of physical debilitation. On top of this the cytotoxic drugs depress the body's natural defence mechanisms, making the patient, while on a course of chemotherapy, much more vulnerable to other infections.

The use of these drugs in addition to surgery is called 'adjuvant chemotherapy' and is designed to mop up any cancerous cells that may have been shed during surgery. There are doctors who believe that by the time a cancerous tumour in the breast is large enough to be felt some cancerous cells will already have shed even when there is no evidence of lymph node involvement. Because cells have shed it does not necessarily mean that they will settle elsewhere and start rapidly multiplying to form a secondary tumour. The body's defences may destroy them before they have a chance to be harmful. Adjuvant chemotherapy is given as a precautionary measure rather than as a form of treatment designed to control known secondary growths. Trials in Italy and America have shown that women given a course of chemotherapy following surgery have had a lower short-term recurrence rate than a control group not given such treatment. Long-term recurrence rates between the two groups are still to be measured.

A course of adjuvant chemotherapy is usually based on a much lower dosage and is given over a period of months. This precautionary (prophylactic) dose gives rise either to fewer or to less unpleasant side-effects. The cytotoxic drugs can be taken orally, but more frequently they are injected or infused directly into the vein over a period of hours. Treatment involves the patient attending hospital out-patients at regular intervals and at each attendance a blood test is done to check, in particular, whether or not the patient is anaemic.

Research is ever ongoing to develop drugs that are effective and which give rise to fewer side-effects. Experiments are also continually under way to improve the combination of drugs used in chemotherapy for it is rare for only one drug to be used. Patients are given a 'cocktail' of cytotoxic drugs, for it is known that some cancer cells are resistant to certain drugs and others develop a resistance. For that reason drugs are combined and combinations are changed, sometimes during a course of treatment.

Despite advances and the lower dosages patients still suffer some side-effects from drugs given as adjuvant therapy. Nausea and fatigue are the most common, but all other side-effects caused by cytotoxic drugs may be suffered. Hair loss can be one of the most distressing. Writing in the *Guardian* on 4 April 1985, Ruth Elliott described the experience of losing her hair while having a course of chemotherapy. Before starting the treatment she asked the doctors, 'Will that mean losing my hair?' and the standard response was 'You may do. Some of it.' Of the attitude of doctors towards hair loss during treatment she wrote:

Many of the much-heralded advances of modern medicine have side-effects which are rarely discussed until they seriously damage or actually kill the patient they're intended to cure. It's all part of the untidiness of human existence that we come in these total packages some parts of which wear out before others. To doctors concerned with halting all this built-in obsolescence, the temporary disappearance of hair is hardly even a side issue.

Or, she might have added the possible temporary cessation of periods.

Besides research into drugs that produce fewer side-effects research has been done into ways of adjusting diets in order to minimize those effects. Professor Kenneth Calman found that cancer patients were invariably short of vitamin A. At the Glasgow hospital where he works he gave patients large doses of vitamin A and found that they responded much better to chemotherapy than those patients with low levels of this vitamin in their blood. If you are having a course of chemotherapy it is worth asking your doctor about this and having a blood test to ascertain your need for a large dose of vitamin A.

Most research into the use of chemotherapy has been aimed at its use as treatment in the advanced stages of the disease or as treatment additional to surgery. Dr Tomlinson at the Mount Vernon Hospital has been looking at the possible use of chemotherapy in some cases as a form of primary treatment in itself or in addition to radiotherapy. The main part of his work has involved carefully measuring tumour growth, believing that this can give vital information as to how a patient should be treated. He believes that this information could avert radical surgery and indicate what sort of lesser surgery is required, or whether chemotherapy or radiotherapy should be used in its place. His work has also included much research into the strength of doses in chemotherapy and the careful monitoring of the drug combinations. On the basis of results so far Dr Tomlinson claims that in the first few years of this form of treatment 'It has been shown statistically, with a high degree of probability, that fewer patients are dying than with standard forms of management.' Unfortunately his research project at the

Mount Vernon Hospital is under threat as the Medical Research Council has refused to provide further funding. It is hoped that other funding will be found so that the research can continue enabling their findings to be properly evaluated.

One of the big reservations about the use of cytotoxic drugs in primary treatment either as adjuvant therapy or as the primary form of treatment itself is that little is known of the long-term effects. Cytotoxic drugs, after all, are toxic (poisonous). While it is known that they affect normal and cancerous cells alike it is also known that healthy cells recover more quickly but the long-term damage to healthy cells and to the body's defence system is not really known. It is also not known whether cytotoxic drugs are, in the long term, in themselves cancer causing. Many of the toxins remain in the body long after treatment has ceased. We should take a long hard look at the effects of the use of cytotoxic drugs.

Like all other forms of treatment for breast cancer, chemotherapy is the subject of fierce debate. There is a wide divergence of opinion about when and whether it should be used, what its effectiveness is and in what dosages and combinations it is best used. It is thought to be of greater value to pre-menopausal than to post-menopausal women.

If a course of chemotherapy is suggested you should ask why, whether there is evidence to make the doctor think that it is necessary, whether it is being suggested as a precautionary measure, whether it could be considered as a primary treatment in itself without surgery or whether it should be 'kept' as a form of treatment in case of recurrence. Before it begins you should also ask how long the course of treatment will take, what side-effects the particular combination of drugs they intend to give are likely to cause, whether you will be able to continue your normal life during treatment and what action you can take to minimize the side-effects and make you less vulnerable to infection, for instance, a course of vitamin A tablets or other dietary measures. Be prepared too for the additional costs of chemotherapy; they can mount up. You don't have to pay for the treatment itself, but you do have to pay the prescription charges for any other drugs you take at home.

Hormone therapy
Hormone therapy is the other weapon in the armoury of orthodox medicine for the treatment of breast cancer. It has usually been considered as an additional treatment at the primary stage, or as a form of treatment to be reserved in case of local recurrence or distant spread. But increasingly it is moving to the front of the stage as a form of treatment. This change has been brought about by much greater insight into the different types of breast cancer and their links with hormonal activity. Recent results from the use of hormone therapy in the form of the drug Tamoxifen have been encouraging enough to make it something to be considered when discussing primary forms of treatment.

It has long been known, indeed since 1896, that women's ovarian secretions - female hormones, particularly oestrogen - are in some way related to breast cancer. Working on this knowledge and on the fact that in some women remission of the disease was achieved for a time following the surgical removal of their ovaries, surgeons adopted a policy of routinely removing a woman's ovaries (oopherectomy) following a mastectomy. This was done 'blind', the surgeons not knowing either why the operation helped some women or which women it would help. The routine use of the operation was eventually dropped by most surgeons who felt they could not justify the physical and emotional trauma caused by the operation, particularly to pre-menopausal women, when they did not know which patients it would benefit.

Recent research, however, has shown which women, with what kinds of breast cancer, would be most likely to respond to hormone therapy, particularly the drug Tamoxifen. It has been found that breast cancers fall into three main categories. These are determined by the levels of tiny molecules called oestrogen receptor protein found in them.

About a third of all breast cancers are strongly oestrogen dependent, one-third are variable oestrogen dependent and

61

another third are oestrogen independent. Women with strongly oestrogen-dependent breast cancers are very likely to respond to some form of hormone therapy, either by means of surgery or of drug therapy and many of those in the grey area are also likely to respond to such treatment. Women with cancers that are strongly oestrogen independent are those who would benefit least or not at all from hormone therapy and would therefore be candidates for other forms of treatment.

With the availability of this information, surgeons should no longer perform surgery to remove the ovaries 'blind' but only for specific patients who indicate a high probability of responding.

While it is perfectly possible to gather the crucial information about oestrogen-dependent or -independent cancers it is rarely done, for it is obtained as a result of a test called an Oestrogen Receptor assay. The American spelling, Estrogen is used. ER assays are *not* available on the NHS and the few women who have one will have it done primarily for research reasons. Rose Krushner, an American who has researched into and written extensively on the subject of breast cancer, argues that *all* women before having their first biopsy should make sure that an ER assay will be done. It must be performed at the time of the first biopsy and prior arrangements must be made as the cancerous tissue to be tested has to be frozen within 15 minutes of its removal from the breast. The results of the ER assay show whether the cancer is oestrogen dependent and, if so, how strongly, or whether it is oestrogen independent. In discussing treatment and before having a biopsy done you should ask whether an ER assay will be done and if the answer is no, which it probably will be, then the next question should be 'Why not?' Only if women demand ER assays will they become accepted as routine and budgeted as part of the health service. Even though it is an expensive test, if it can lead to effective and cheaper long-term treatment, then its cost is more than justified.

The need for more information about the ER status of breast cancers and their response to hormone therapy is confirmed by a report published in the *Lancet* (13 April 1985). The report gives the findings of a 'controlled trial' on the use of Tamoxifen as the sole additional treatment given to patients who had early breast cancer. It found, after monitoring for six years 1,285 patients aged 75 or less, who were part of the trial and who were put at random (one hopes with their fully informed consent) into a Tamoxifen treated group and a control group, that:

There has been a significant prolongation of the disease-free interval in the Tamoxifen treated group followed by a highly significant reduction in death rate, with 45 (34 per cent) fewer deaths observed in the treated group than in the control group. This benefit appeared to be independent of menopausal, nodal, or ER status.

These findings should, as the report points out, be interpreted cautiously. Some of the patients in the trial have not been observed for long, the most recent of them having had only one year of Tamoxifen, the trial period being for up to two years of treatment. The report concludes that 'This is the first trial demonstrating a significant survival benefit with Tamoxifen and we hope for confirmation of this important effect in other trials of similar design currently in progress.'

Given the assertion, despite the plea for cautious interpretation, that Tamoxifen is beneficial to a significant group of women, one is again left with the question about controlled trials based on randomized selection. When the benefits of Tamoxifen are now clearly thought to be significant it hardly seems ethical to withhold it from some women for the sake of randomized controlled trials. Other ways of monitoring its benefit should be devised.

This trial is also the first to have monitored the side-effects of Tamoxifen which previously had not been very well charted. Only 25 patients (4 per cent) of those on Tamoxifen discontinued it because of its unwanted side-effects. Other patients reported a variety of side-effects, although it is still not clear how many of those can be attributed to Tamoxifen and how many to other causes. Since Tamoxifen works as an oestrogen blocker the main side-effect is to bring about the menopause. The speed with which this happens is uncertain and seems to vary greatly. For women who have had the menopause this is a side-effect which obviously does not concern them. Nor does it much concern women who are approaching the menopause or who are sure that they do not want either to have, or to have any more, children. It is obviously a serious side-effect for any woman who wants a child.

Other side-effects of Tamoxifen are hot flushes, sometimes with profuse sweating. Women taking it have also complained about skin rashes, headaches, which can be severe, nausea, tiredness and, very commonly, depression. In the case of depression it is often hard to work out whether it is caused by the drug itself or whether it is an understandable reaction to a daily dose which reminds the patient that they have had or have breast cancer. Some women who have stopped taking Tamoxifen have commented how much 'better' physically and emotionally they felt, confirming the suspicion that for some Tamoxifen is a depressive drug.

Many of the women we have spoken to have taken or are taking Tamoxifen. It is taken regularly, one pill a day, either as a precautionary measure or as a direct form of treatment for recurrence or distant spread. Jill Louw had local recurrence in the breast in which she had a primary tumour some five years ago. Following the biopsy she started taking Tamoxifen. Within a month the lump had shrunk considerably and continues to shrink. Another woman we interviewed who had secondary growths in her ribs and spine found that Tamoxifen was causing them to shrink and in some cases to disappear altogether. She, like Jill, is having no other form of treatment. Another woman interviewed in a video about breast cancer called *Why Me?* who had breast cancer and distant spread had been treated with Tamoxifen only and after some months on the drug she too reported that she felt much better and there were signs of her breast tumour shrinking. While Tamoxifen is increasingly used with good effect, it is a drug about which we still have little information. Its long-term effects are unknown and it will be some time before they are recognized.

The use of Tamoxifen as a preventive measure is also being considered particularly for post-menopausal women. The Imperial Cancer Research Fund is hoping to raise the money to undertake a seven-year trial involving 4,000 women to see whether Tamoxifen taken as a preventive measure will, in fact, reduce the incidence of breast cancer. The trial will be based on giving one group of women Tamoxifen over a period of five to seven years and comparing their incidence of breast cancer with a control group who would not have taken the drug as a preventive measure. The theory behind the trial being that since many breast cancers are oestrogen dependent, the amount of oestrogen in the bloodstream will govern the growth of oestrogen-dependent cancers. This theory is based on the initial results of the trials of Tamoxifen in the treatment of breast cancer. In the light of the questionable track record of such trials one can only hope that any women participating in this proposed trial will consent to do so only if they are really informed.

It is too soon really to hope that Tamoxifen is a major breakthrough in the treatment of breast cancer for some women, but the initial signs are positive. Hence you should ask if it is a possible primary form of treatment. It is not easy to argue for a biopsy and an ER assay before any other form of treatment is considered when confronted by a consultant who almost certainly is suggesting surgery, but to do so may well be worthwhile in the long term.

Should I get a second opinion?

The list of questions patients shall ask their doctors compiled by the US Department of Health and Human Services includes, 'Should I get an opinion from another doctor?' In three episodes of the American TV policewoman series *Cagney and Lacey* Lacey had clearly not read the pamphlet, her colleague Cagney probably had. Lacey's first surgeon advised her, after her lump had been diagnosed as malignant, to have a mastectomy which would include the removal of her lymph glands. Between fighting crime Cagney tried to persuade Lacey to get a second opinion. The audience was kept on tenterhooks while Lacey at first rejected the idea of going elsewhere but then agreed. Much to Lacey's, and the audience's, relief the second surgeon advised different treatment. Based on the size of her lump, less than two centimetres, and its position, the outer quadrant, he suggested that she only needed a lumpectomy and that during surgery a biopsy of the lymph nodes could be performed to see if they were involved.

When the findings were available the second surgeon suggested that radiotherapy might be wise but dismissed the previous doctor's opinion that surgery would have to be followed by chemotherapy. Lacey opted to follow the advice gained from the second surgeon who reassured her that with the type and size of her lump her long-term outlook would be at least as good as if she had had more extensive surgery. The moral of these episodes of *Cagney and Lacey* was clearly 'Get a second opinion'.

Asking for a second opinion seems, on the face of it, like a perfectly reasonable request. Why, then, is it so rarely asked of British doctors? Why, too, do British doctors so rarely suggest that a second opinion should be sought? Usually such a suggestion is only made in extremely rare or complicated cases. Breast cancer is neither rare nor is its treatment thought to be medically complicated. Most surgeons appear to be certain that what they advise is the best possible known treatment, and confronted with such an appearance of certainty patients rarely question it. But breast cancer is a supreme example of a field of medicine in which opinions should be questioned and second opinions sought.

This is the case because of the wide divergences of opinion about treatments and because of the wide range of attitudes and practices among the medical practitioners themselves. This divergence was highlighted by a survey done by S.M. Gore and colleagues of *Treatment Decisions in Breast Cancer*. The research team created two fictitious women called Mrs Martin and Mrs O'Neill. Both were in their early fifties with a 4cm cancerous tumour but different lymph node involvement and receptor status. They then asked doctors in Scotland and Australia what treatments they would give to these two women. 62 doctors replied as to how they would treat Mrs Martin and they presented 36 different plans for treatment. There was proportionally an even greater number of opinions about how to treat Mrs O'Neill. 52 doctors replied giving 42 different plans. Clearly a woman can get almost as many different opinions about the best possible combination of treatments as the number of doctors she consults. Caught up in this debate is the individual patient referred to a particular surgeon and subject to her or his opinion or preference. So you may quite arbitrarily find yourself treated by a surgeon who believes in mastectomy followed by radiotherapy, or one who goes for lumpectomies, radiotherapy and chemotherapy, or one who offers implants, or one who suggests hormone therapy as primary treatment. You may find yourself with the rare surgeon who is willing to explore complementary therapies or you may be with one who will virtually refuse to treat you if you so much as swallow a glass of carrot juice. Because of this it is most important that you feel that you have the right to seek a second opinion. But few of us feel, or know, we have that right, or if we do, have the nerve to pursue it. In America you pay for treatment and this makes it easier for those who have the cash to seek a second opinion. Getting a second opinion from the NHS is free, but many patients in the NHS do not know how to get one.

In Britain it is easier for an out-patient than for an in-patient to get a second opinion. Once inside a hospital, as one woman put it, 'they've got you by the short and curlies'. Initially your GP refers you to a surgeon whom either you choose or who is his or her recommendation (see the section on first referral). If after a consultation with that surgeon you are for any reason unhappy and want a second opinion or merely to see someone with whom you may be able to communicate better, then you should go back to your GP. Explain your reasons for wanting a second opinion and ask your GP to write another letter to another consultant (preferably at a different hospital), explaining that the referral is for a second opinion. Before doing this it is wise to ask around to find out which consultant would be best. This is difficult but it can either be done by talking to other women who have had breast cancer or by contacting relevant organizations. However, when contacting organizations it is worth checking out their attitudes. For instance the Mastectomy Association is not likely to be the organization best equipped to tell you the name and place of a consultant who offers to do lumpectomies.

Most surgeons respond positively to patients who have gone to them for a second opinion. Simply asking for a second opinion shows the patient to be a discriminating consumer and the surgeon realizes that he or she is under question. This usually acts in the patient's favour and he or she is treated with a little more respect than is usually the case.

If after getting a second opinion you want to go back to the first consultant, there is no reason why you should not do so. The first consultant need never know that you have been elsewhere. This may seem as if you are protecting the consultant's feelings but many patients fear that if they question their consultant's opinion openly then the way they are subsequently treated will be affected.

This fear is particularly acute for an in-patient. It is extremely hard, when one cannot use a third party – the GP, to say to the white-coated figure by your bed, 'I would like a second opinion.' One assumes that it would immediately be interpreted as a doubt about his or her medical competence. Most patients respect, rather than lose confidence in, a doctor who either accepts the need for, or suggests a second opinion. If as an in-patient you are seriously concerned about the treatment offered to you, you can contact your GP, get a friend or relative to ask for a second opinion or discharge yourself and then ask your GP to refer you elsewhere. This last course of action is a difficult and dramatic one to take, but, ultimately, if it leads you to a form of treatment which you find acceptable then your feelings not those of the surgeons are the ones to be considered.

In almost all other fields second opinions are normal but the practice is far from accepted in medicine. The sooner it is, the better it will be for the patient and the better for the doctor. Doctors will no longer need to play God and can be mortal with skills that we respect but also with recognizable preferences and fallibilities which do not make them any the less doctors. The patient–doctor relationship could then be based on mutual respect.

As will be evident the answer to this question posed in this section has been phrased here entirely in terms of orthodox medicine. You may well want a second opinion from alternative medicine, but there is little point in asking the average orthodox practitioner whether they advise doing so. For opinions and second opinions within alternative medicine you will have to ask the practitioners in that field.

Can I see a nurse counsellor?

In some hospitals the answer will be yes, in some a talk with the nurse counsellor will have been offered to you before you even ask, but in most hospitals the answer will be 'No, we don't have one.' Nurse counsellors are relatively new in the treatment of breast cancer patients. It may have seemed blatantly obvious to the thousands and thousands of women who have had and have breast cancer that there is a need for them to talk to someone. That need, until recently, has not been officially recognized.

It has been due particularly to the work of Dr Peter Maguire, a senior lecturer in psychiatry at the University Hospital of South Machester, that this need has not only been recognized but acted upon. His work on the psychological and social consequences of breast cancer has shown doctors that women facing breast cancer suffer from a very high level of anxiety which is barely acknowledged. Writing of his research in the *Nursing Mirror* in 1975 Dr Maguire commented, 'While surgeons and nurses had expected that some women would be worried by their lumps, they seriously underestimated the true number.' The reasons for this were found in the failures of communication between medical staff and patients. Medical staff, it was found, all too frequently failed to pick up and respond to the verbal and non-verbal distress signals that women gave out. The women themselves hid their true feelings particularly from the surgeons.

This reluctance by women to tell their surgeons how they felt, apart from their physical health, was explained thus: 'they were afraid that they might look silly, that they did not want to overburden the staff who, they knew, were already busy, and that it was inappropriate to take their worries to people who were primarily concerned with patients physical health'.

In order that women should have someone with whom they feel it is appropriate to discuss their worries, nurse counsellors came into being, sadly all too slowly. More than a decade after the publication of Dr Peter Maguire's research nurse counsellors are employed only in a minority of breast units. Asking this question may help to make them a standard part of every breast unit team. Enough demand might create sufficient supply.

The nurse counsellor's role is to offer emotional and practical support to the patient. She is primarily the patient's friend, someone with time, with understanding and whose face doesn't change with changing duty rosters. Unlike other medical staff she is not tied to one place and can see you at the clinic, in the ward, at home or be available at the end of a telephone line. Sylvia Denton, the nurse counsellor in the King's College Hospital Breast Unit, described the nurse counsellor's role:

> With sufficient tact and a modicum of skill a relationship may be rapidly established between the patient and her nurse, enabling her to express her doubts and fears and to explore possible solutions to her problems. Knowledge of current treatment of breast cancer, together with information regarding prosthesis, clothing and provision for care within other agencies, such as the social services, charities and other medical disciplines, is essential before a nurse attempts counselling. This knowledge should extend to the services provided within the community, for it is only when the patient emerges from the hospital gates upon discharge that she faces the realities of life again without the 'cocoon' of the hospital and the supportive 'feminine' environment of the ward.

The nurse counsellor is most importantly there as someone with whom you can discuss 'doubts and fears', but as can be seen from Sylvia Denton's 'job description' the nurse counsellor can provide much more. As a person well informed about breast cancer she is able to explain things and discuss different forms of treatment. All too frequently a patient emerges from a consultation with a doctor/surgeon bewildered, unclear as to what was said and too traumatized or intimidated to ask any questions. To have someone who can go over an explanation with you slowly so that you understand clearly is invaluable. The unasked questions can be asked, the admission of ignorance can be made and because the relationship is with a woman other questions can be asked that many women would feel embarrassed to ask of a male doctor.

A nurse counsellor should make sure no woman is sent home following a mastectomy being told, when she asked about a prosthesis, to roll up her knickers and stuff them in her bra (see the interview with Jenny on p. 128). Likewise no woman who has access to a nurse counsellor should remain ignorant of the exercises that can be done following surgery to help get back mobility. But it is the continuation of counselling after a patient has left hospital or while an out-patient that is perhaps one of their most important roles. The social and psychological problems of breast cancer are very great. Dr Peter Maguire found a high level of anxiety, depression (sometimes verging on suicidal depression), marital stress and social problems in women who had breast cancer. Even the strongest of marriages and relationships are put under stress by the fact of one partner having cancer and being physically changed. In marriages already under stress breast cancer can be the breaking point.

The fact of having breast cancer changes a woman both emotionally and physically and that change has to be confronted both by the woman herself and by those around her. The process can be painful and difficult to live with and to live through. One husband described his wife's reaction to Dr Maguire.

She was very depressed. In fact, to express the extent to which she was depressed, I had some very trying times. She believed everybody was against her. At two in the morning I'd have to get up and reassure her that I wanted her, the family wanted her . . . She slept on her own . . . She went into the spare bedroom. I couldn't make this out . . . she's more or less renounced our married life recently, and for more or less a week she didn't want to have anything to do with anybody . . . I had to stop her from more or less retreating into a world of her own . . . She was saying that she'd had enough of life and would be better off without it.

That wife's reaction was not uncommon. Not surprisingly many women have 'sexual problems' following a mastectomy. It is hard for a woman in our society of 'page 3' tits, Dolly Parton jokes, of colour supplement physical perfection and female bodies displayed all over the place as sex objects to come to terms with a body which, as the poet Erike Mumford wrote after having had a mastectomy, is 'half woman and half eunuch'. Breasts are part of our identity as women, part of our femaleness and our femininity. To lose one, and sometimes two, is to feel the loss of part of that identity. To be able to grieve over that loss and come to terms with it is difficult. It is much easier if one is loved, supported and understood. Talking about those feelings also can help. Many women don't have anyone to talk to and a nurse counsellor is there precisely to listen.

All women who have had cancer have to learn to live with the fear that it may return. It is learning to live with that fear in every ache, pain, sore throat or slightest change in the breast. It is learning to live with the fear that, despite whatever treatment, some cancerous cells are lurking somewhere in the body waiting to strike at any time. It is learning to live with the fear of death as a reality rather than something that happens to us all 'one day'. The taboos about cancer, talking about it, admitting to having it still run deep. But to be silent about it is often to leave the person most in need, the cancer patient, frightened and isolated. A nurse counsellor cannot magic away all these fears but she can help by being a sympathetic listener.

Obviously since the relationship with a nurse counsellor is one-to-one not all patients will find a rapport with their nurse counsellor, but all patients with access to a nurse counsellor should find that they benefit at least from the practical point of view. If the rapport is not such that the patient feels she can discuss other worries and fears, then the nurse counsellor can direct the patient to other support groups which may help. Nurse counsellors can also, as the central link with the patient, sometimes bridge the warring camps of orthodox and alternative medicine. They can discuss with patients relaxation techniques and their benefit, dietary changes and other changes in life-style. They can feed back to the medical staff a better insight into patients' feelings. To do just this a four-year study of mastectomy patients and their post-operative feelings has been conducted. Joan Anderson who is analysing the data hopes that 'the project will let us understand the woman's viewpoint and the ways in which we can be more helpful'. The doctors, she adds, are primarily concerned with the patient's diseased body and therefore fail to listen 'to patients and self-help groups which are there because the professionals are not meeting human need nor recognizing patient priorities' (*Guardian*, 18 July 1985). Nurse counsellors are a step forward towards meeting that human need but while surgeons can still tell a woman that he intends removing her breast simply by putting an 'x' mark on her diseased breast then there is still a long way to go in understanding the woman's viewpoint.

8. Non-cancerous breast disorders

The Structure and Function of the Breast

> They said it was infected milk ducts that had caused the
> lump. I couldn't understand it. I didn't understand what
> that means. They never showed me a picture or really
> explained how the breast functioned. They didn't
> understand how this lump had formed but that was the
> explanation I got when I left the hospital.
>
> (Ann)

A very high percentage of women experience, at some time in
their lives, some kind of disorder of the breast. Disorders range
from tenderness just before a period to recurrent cysts, persistent
pain, discharge and infections. These all arise from the structure
of the breast and its function of producing milk. The key
element therefore (see Diagram I p.37) of the breast which
develops during puberty is its milk production system. The
production line starts in the breast lobules where the milk is
produced. It then passes through small ducts to reservoirs
beneath the nipple where it is collected ready for the baby to
draw from when it sucks the nipple. The milk is sucked out
through small ducts in the nipple. For most of women's adult
lives these days milk is not being produced though the system is
in a continual state of readiness between puberty and the
menopause.

Between this central milk production network there is a lot of
glandular and fibrous tissue separating the milk channels and
giving the breast shape and support. In the breast too there are

also nerves, fat, arteries, veins, lymphatic channels and connective tissue all there to serve and support the main function of
the breast. It is not surprising that things can go wrong in this
sensitive system with many elements, particularly since the
system is continually reacting to changes signalled by hormones.
During every menstrual cycle the breast, like the womb,
responds to hormones and prepares for a possible pregnancy.
Prior to ovulation, that is, during the first two weeks of a
monthly cycle, the milk ducts in the breast and the supporting
fibrous tissue grow. After the egg is released the milk glands
swell with fluid in preparation for milk production. If a
pregnancy does not occur, the accumulated fluid and tissues are
broken down by special cells of the lymph's system then drained
from the breast into the body. At the menopause this process
stops, the glandular tissue slowly atrophies and is replaced by
fatty tissue, though some women can retain quite a lot of their
ducts and glandular tissue into old age.

Throughout a woman's life her breasts are constantly
changing. Because of this it is sometimes hard for a woman, or
even for a doctor, to decide where the changes are normal or
signs of abnormality. The monthly feeling of fullness just before
a period is normal, though it becomes abnormal if that fullness
changes from tenderness to pain and is accompanied by a lump
or lumpiness. A tiny amount of clear fluid discharge from both
nipples which often goes unnoticed is normal, but a coloured or
bloody discharge or a discharge from one duct in one nipple can
often signify abnormality. A condition called fibrosis (thickening) is both normal and abnormal. It is part of the natural
process of ageing after the menopause when fibrous tissue takes
over the tissue that had been part of the milk production system.
In younger women this process of thickening can happen
though it usually happens in particular areas of the breast rather
than in the breast generally as in the post-menopausal woman.
Women who have suffered a rapid weight loss for one reason or
another can find that their breasts feel abnormal, lumpy or full
of thickened tissue. This feeling can be brought about by the
rapid weight loss itself and by the change in the breast's tissue.

Protruding as they do, women's breasts are prone to bump into things or be bumped into. There is no evidence that such normal daily 'wear and tear' does them any harm. It is only through severe injury that tissue in the breast is damaged. Fortunately, given all the other things that can go wrong with the breasts we cannot break any bones or strain any muscles in them for they have neither. There are basically no muscles within the breast itself, but there are muscles behind the breast on the chest wall (the *pectoralis major*), muscles just above the breast and below the shoulder blade (the *pectoralis minor*) and other muscles surrounding the breast on the side of the body and in the upper arm.

Since doctors often have considerable difficulty in describing and explaining in language comprehensible to the lay person what is wrong with them, it is surprising that they do not routinely use visual aids to assist their explanations. It would cost little and would greatly help women to understand if all breast units had large clear section drawings or even section models of the breast. For instance, a woman complaining of discharge and told she has a 'duct papilloma' is most unlikely, unless she has a medical training or is well read on the subject, to have a clue what the doctor is talking about. If that woman can be shown a diagram of where the duct is (the papillomas usually occur in the lactiferous ducts – Diagram I) and see how that duct is connected to the ducts in the nipple then she will at least get a picture of where the trouble is. If this is accompanied by the explanation that a papilloma is a small warty type of growth in the duct and that it is causing the yellowish or possibly bloody discharge from her nipple, then the fog is likely to clear and she will not only get a picture of where and what it is but also an understanding of it.

Perhaps as women we should know how our breasts are structured but for most of us our education included only rudimentary biology. So if you don't understand where in your breast the disorder is, it is worth asking to be shown on a drawing or diagram. Enough demand for diagrams might lead to their permanent use as a routine part of explanation.

NON-CANCEROUS BREAST DISORDERS

What breast disorder do I have?

During those three months I continued to get discharge
intermittently. I also got considerable pain on the left side
of my breast. The pain came and went at no particular time
and was quite different from the general tenderness I feel
in my breasts just before a period. On my return visit to
the hospital for a check-up, I decided to ask what my
symptoms were. I particularly wanted to know if the
symptoms could be an indication of a pre-cancerous state.
My asking 'What is wrong with me?' elicited the response
'You really shouldn't worry, nothing is wrong with you',
and by implication it was clear that the doctor thought I
was a neurotic woman worrying about nothing. Pathetically
I said, 'Well, I'd just like to know', and in response the
doctor said that if I was really worried they would do me a
big favour and see me again in three months.

(Sarah)

Asking for your breast disorder to be named is not always, for
a variety of reasons, the simple question it appears to be. It is not
simple in some cases because although doctors know of the
symptoms, hearing about them regularly in clinics, they are
unsure of the causes. In other cases there is confusion in the
terms used to describe the various conditions probably because
there is confusion about the conditions themselves. Some
professionals writing about the breast use their own terminology
as if it were *the* accepted terminology, ignoring the fact that
other doctors use other words. Professor Baum comments that:

There is still considerable confusion amongst the lay
public, the ancillary professions, and amongst doctors
themselves as to the precise meaning of the terms that are
commonly used in relation to diseases of the breast. For
example, such simple words as tumour, lesion, benign and
malignant are commonly tossed around by doctors in such
a way to confuse themselves, let alone their patients.

The word tumour as he rightly points out merely means 'a swelling' and a *benign* tumour is a swelling that does not spread to other parts of the body. It may cause discomfort or pain but it is almost never life threatening. A *malignant* tumour is a cancerous tumour.

If there is confusion about the 'simple' words describing breast diseases, there is even more confusion in the use of names for non-cancerous breast disorders. Nowhere is the confusion greater than in what is generally known as cystic breast disease.

What is cystic breast disease?

If you have painfully swollen and lumpy breasts or a single, usually tender lump (a cyst), then your condition is called cystic breast disease. It may, however, also be called mastitis, cystic mastitis and fibrocystic disease. To confuse the issue further mastitis is also used to describe a condition usually only suffered during breast-feeding. This type of mastitis is an inflammation of the breast caused by a blocked duct and should not be confused with cystic breast disease, since its causes and its treatments are quite different.

Cystic breast disease probably has so many names as it is the commonest of all breast disorders. It is estimated that about half of all women suffer from it at one time or another. For many the symptoms are temporary, emerging for two or three months and then disappearing. They can just be a small accentuation of the normal feelings of change during the monthly cycle or they can be extreme. For other women the symptoms come month after month, year after year causing discomfort, pain and distress. Tied as women's bodies are to cycles it has been noticed that this condition tends to be at its worst for women living in the northern hemisphere when their ovaries are most active during the months of December to May. It also affects the left breast more than the right; almost twice as many women complain of pain in their left breast than in their right or both.

Cystic disease is caused either by the breasts preparing for milk production too enthusiastically during the first half of the monthly cycle and/or failing to drain properly or blocking the accumulated fluid during the second half of the cycle. This production of excess fluid and the failure to drain it away properly causes the swelling. In some women the blockages can lead to the growth of one or more large fluid filled cysts and in others to the growth of numerous small cysts. 'Cure' for this condition usually comes with the menopause when with the cessation of the menstrual cycle the breasts stop their monthly cycle of preparation for milk production. While being pleased that the menopause will bring an end to such symptoms many women feel they cannot wait, maybe for years, before they get relief. Those with distinct lumps particularly wish to look both for treatment and for reassurance that they do not have cancer. Those with pain wish for pain relief, particularly when it is severe enough to cause sleepless nights as well.

What treatments are there for cystic breast disease?

Asking me about the amount of pain, discomfort and worry I had, he offered me a choice of three forms of treatment, explaining the pros and cons of each. I could have surgery but that, in his experience, was not usually very successful and that I would, as likely as not, return a year later with the same symptoms. I could have hormone treatment, but that had side-effects, or we could 'just wait and see'.

(Sarah)

No one treatment has been found safe and totally successful for this condition. Treatments vary partially in relation to the severity and frequency of the symptoms and partially in relation to the preferences of the doctor prescribing the treatment. Curiously this is one area of treatment for breast disorders where orthodox medicine and alternative medicine are not entirely at loggerheads. Orthodox researchers, besides trying to develop drugs, have also looked at treating cystic breast disease by giving large doses of Vitamin E and also through dietary changes. Women have to weigh their symptoms, their severity and the

79

distress they cause against the risk of different forms of treatment. In this instance, since the disorder is persistent a woman can choose complementary alternative treatment alongside some orthodox treatments and see which works best for her. Recent research in the USA has shown that certain dietary changes can lead to a reduction or even cessation of the symptoms of cystic breast disease. Dr Minton of the Ohio State University in his researches found a connection between a group of chemicals known as methylxanthines and the disease. These chemicals are found in tea, coffee, cocoa and in certain 'fizzy' drinks like Coca Cola and Pepsi. Dr Minton found that in a group of 120 women with cystic breast disease who eliminated methylxanthines from their diet 80 had their cysts gradually disappear. These women remained clear of their condition as long as they followed their diet. Although this 'treatment' has not had widespread testing it has been enough to impress other doctors who have suggested it to their patients. The results of Dr Minton's researches would make it seem worthwhile for any woman with cystic breast disease to try this form of treatment. After all it is safe and involves only minimal dietary changes. The exception may be those women who have a single distinct cyst and who fear that it may be cancer and want it investigated as well as changing their diet. Indeed some doctors in the USA are now recommending trying the removal of methylzanthines from the diet first; if that fails, hormone treatment can be tried.

Another treatment that is being tried in the USA and has also achieved a measure of success in reducing or curing the disorder is large doses of Vitamin E given daily over a period of eight weeks. This treatment has as yet only undergone preliminary testing and it is not known what the long term side-effects may be of taking a course of such high doses of Vitamin E. Women may well feel that a two-month course of megadoses of Vitamin E would be less risky with fewer side effects both in the short term and the long term than taking a course of conventional drug treatment.

A third treatment is in the form of a drug called Danazol. It is made from the synthetic hormone danocrine and reduces breast pain, lumpiness and tenderness in a high percentage of the women who take it. The drug is usually given for a period of six months during which a variety of side-effects may be felt. It can cause weight gain, facial hair growth, water retention and irregular periods or period loss. These side-effects stop at the end of the course of treatment and for most women the beneficial effects of the drug last for up to two years. Although the drug has been, as they say, 'rigorously tested', women would be wise to be wary of such hormone-based treatments. Little is known of the long-term effects. If your doctor suggests a course of hormone treatment it is worth asking about the long- and short-term side-effects and weighing them against the severity of your symptoms.

A woman with a distinct lump would be wise to get it treated or analysed. This kind of lump or cyst is usually filled with a watery fluid. Sometimes it grows, becomes tender and then reduces of its own accord without any treatment. Others grow and stay, often causing considerable pain. Those that do not drain away themselves can be treated by needle aspiration (see section on needle aspiration). This usually gives almost instant physical relief and it can give mental relief since, as a precaution, some of the fluid is always sent away for analysis. This condition can and does recur and so if you get cysts it would be worth trying dietary changes in order to try to stop them. Surgery should not be necessary for this condition and if your surgeon suggests it, it would be worth asking if it is really necessary. While surgical removal of cysts does take place in this country, although less frequently than it did, more radical surgery has not been tried. It has been known for women in the USA who suffer from severe, recurrent cystic disease to have all the breast tissue under the skin removed surgically and to have a synthetic implant to replace it. It is a form of treatment hardly to be recommended for while it removes the source of the problem, the breast, it replaces it with another, a silicone implant, not to mention the risk from and side-effects of surgery.

The future for women with cystic breast disease does seem to be hopeful. New treatments based on dietary changes and vitamin supplements, if successful, will mean an end to suffering, discomfort and distress for many women with few, if any, risky side-effects.

What are the other common and uncommon breast disorders?

Non-cancerous tumours occur in the breast. 'Oma' is added to the end of the word which describes where in the breast the growth is sited. A duct papilloma is a small growth in the ducts, a fibroadenoma would be located in the fibrous, glandular tissues of the breast and lipoma in the connective tissues. The most common is the fibroadenoma, which is the second most common breast disease after cystic breast disease. Unlike cancer it occurs more frequently in young women than in older women and can occur in teenage girls. A fibroadenoma or 'a lump', as most women would describe it, feels firm, even solid, but unlike cancerous lumps it is very mobile and difficult to feel. Their size can vary from one to five centimetres in diameter and they tend to grow very slowly. With such a lump you will probably, almost certainly, have been referred to a hospital and as with all lumps you will be fearful as to its nature. From the feel of a fibroadenoma doctors can usually confidently diagnose it. The treatment for such lumps is almost universally standard – surgical removal. This involves a few days in hospital, a general anaesthetic, a small incision, the actual removal of the lump and the resultant small scar. There is no real reason why the fibroadenoma should be removed, for as far as it is known they do not become malignant if untreated. If it grows large it can become disfiguring and a woman may well then feel she wants it removed or it may be wise to remove it while it is still small. Removing the lump also removes the worry of having a lump, even one that is benign.

Lipomas are similar to fibroadenomas except that they are lumps composed of fatty tissue. They can occur anywhere in the body and the breast is no exception. They often do not show up on X-rays but they can usually be felt. A lipoma, like a fibroadenoma, is of no danger but it too may grow large and be disfiguring. For the same reasons it is also treated by surgery requiring as with a fibroadenoma a few days in hospital, a general anaesthetic and minor surgery.

Unlike the other two, a duct papilloma is thought to be, in some cases, a pre-cancerous condition. Its main symptom is a discharge. This should not be confused with the very small discharge from both nipples that comes from the normal workings of the breast. The discharge caused by a duct papilloma usually comes from one duct in one nipple and may be watery, bloody or even greenish. If discharge particularly of this description is your symptom then a duct papilloma is what your surgeon will be looking for. A small amount of discharge will be sent for analysis to check whether it is cancerous. In looking for a duct papilloma the doctor, usually a surgeon, will feel all around the nipple, pressing on each section. If discharge occurs when a specific section is pressed that indicates the place where the papilloma is. A papilloma being a small warty growth. Some women have no pain with this condition but others do feel a fullness or pain in the nipple area which is relieved when the discharge is expressed.

Doctors vary in their attitude as to whether the papilloma should be removed or not. Although not a major operation the removal of the ducts under the nipple is a tricky one. It involves cutting around part of the areola (brown skin surrounding the nipple), turning that skin back like a flap, finding and removing the papilloma (possibly finding and removing other papillomas and duct disease at the same time) and then stitching it back. The reason given for treating this condition with surgery is that it is suspected of being a pre-cancerous condition and therefore, the argument goes, it is better to remove a possible source of cancerous growth. One of the main problems of surgery for this condition is that once you have had one duct papilloma you are more likely than other women to get another. Fortunately duct papillomas are not very common and duct ectasia is even less common, in fact it is quite rare.

Duct ectasia mainly happens to women over 40 and is caused

by the duct system becoming distended and breaking down. As with duct papilloma the main symptom is a sticky and multi-coloured discharge coming from many ducts in one or both nipples. Besides discharge women also frequently get a burning pain around the nipple and sometimes little swellings can be felt under the skin in the nipple area. In the advanced stage of this condition the situation reverses for as the ducts shrivel up and become fibrous they shorten thus pulling the nipple inwards.

As with the other conditions mentioned in this section, surgery is also the form of treatment offered. However, in the other conditions the surgical treatment involves only minor surgery, the treatment of duct ectasia involves much more extensive surgery. Surgical treatment involves removing most of the breast tissue under the skin and nipple, hence reconstruction is often suggested. Breast reconstruction is not without its problems (see section on breast reconstruction) and women, fortunately only the very few who get this condition, should think very hard before submitting themselves to such major surgery for what is almost certainly not a pre-cancerous condition. As with so many medical dilemmas for women this one is a choice of evils in the absence of any simple, safe treatment.

If I have a non-cancerous breast disorder am I more likely to get breast cancer?

The general consensus is that women with benign breast disease do run an increased risk of getting breast cancer. Until recently in Britain this opinion has been based more on assumption and on research conducted in other countries. However, the findings of a study of women with benign breast disease were published in the *British Medical Journal* in 1984 showing that the study had found that 'Women with a past history of benign breast disease have a slightly increased risk of breast cancer.'

This study was based on following up 791 women who had attended diagnostic breast clinics in Wales between 1967 and 1970 and who had, on their first visit during that period, been free of breast cancer. They reported, 'Of the 770 (97 per cent) successfully traced, 22 had developed breast cancer. Based on data available from the Welsh Cancer Registry only 8 cases of breast cancer had been expected, so that the excess risk for the group was 2.7.' The group most at risk were those with cystic breast disease, a finding which was not new but merely confirmed the findings of other studies. While this particular group were the most at risk the study also found that the risk of breast cancer increased for *all* the women, both those who had been found to be 'essentially normal' at their first visit to the clinic as well as those who were found to have some definite breast disease. Of this report it states, 'We, also, however report a new finding: women who attended a breast clinic because of symptoms but who did not have a definite abnormality were also at an increased risk of subsequent breast cancer.' This is an extremely worrying finding in that the conclusion one draws is that attending a breast clinic marginally increases your risk of breast cancer.

Since there is no evidence that cancer is 'caught' like a cold the question arises from these findings as to what happens to women who attend a breast clinic that increases their risk and whether the answer is in the difference between the types of women likely to go to a breast clinic and those who are not. The report hints at some possible answers to these questions and implicitly points to the need for further research.

Despite the greater incidence of breast cancer, women attending the breast clinic were found in this study to have a lower overall mortality rate which, as the report comments, implies that 'they were "healthier" than women in the general population'. It also implies that they were of a higher social class, mortality figures being related to class. Breast cancer statistics are also related to class, the incidence being slightly higher in more affluent social classes. So the class of women studied might have had some bearing on their increased risk but it cannot provide the whole answer.

The report itself admitted, 'We cannot explain our findings', but then goes on to highlight one finding, namely, that there was a very high biopsy rate amongst this particular group of women. In fact they found the biopsy rate was five times higher than expected although 'its predictive value was only 20 per cent'. From that one concludes that biopsies were done when there seemed little need for them. The researchers did not look to see whether this high biopsy rate was a reflection of the individual preferences of the surgeons involved or because of the demands of the women patients. Whatever the reason, this finding must place a question mark over the use of biopsies except when there is a real ground for their need. Clearly further research should have been done following up women who have had biopsies to answer the questions raised by this study. One other aspect that the study did not look at was how many women in the group had a mammogram and how many times.

There is nothing conclusive in this report and its findings but it does tend to confirm the suspicion many of us have that hospitals are 'dangerous places'. Suspicions apart, women should not be deterred from attending a breast clinic because of the findings of this one report. However, they do suggest that women should be wary about diagnostic procedures, agreeing only to those which are felt to be absolutely necessary.

9. Life after treatment

Emotional adjustments

> Someone said you'll have to come in for some tests and you'll need radiotherapy. 'Right,' I said, 'fine', and finally I went home and waited to die basically.
>
> (Jo)

> I coped with my life. I got it right. My way of coping with it was to say, 'Right, I'm in charge now and I'm not going to be put upon.' Although I don't keep to it, every now and again I come back to it.
>
> (Hazel)

A woman treated for breast cancer and then resuming her 'normal' life will have many physical and emotional adjustments to make. The initial period of adjustment can be helped greatly if there is access to a nurse counsellor (see the section on nurse counsellors) and/or if she has strong support systems of her own – husband, lover, relatives, friends. Many women do not have any of these and find themselves discharged at the end of treatment to face the struggle of emotional and physical rehabilitation with no professional support and sometimes little personal support either.

Dealing with the physical problems following surgery is much easier than dealing with the emotional problems. For those women who have had a breast removed they have to deal with their own bereavement. Loss of part of your body is a bereavement. Grieving for part of your lost self takes time and often involves different stages. It is not uncommon for women to come home from hospital feeling that they have 'coped' much better than they anticipated, only to be plunged into deep depression, have violent swings of mood, to be overwhelmed by feelings of anger and outrage or even feel suicidal. All these feelings are not unusual nor do they mean you are in some way unnatural. Working through bereavement is hard and there are no short-cuts but most women with support and help from those close to them and from professionals can work through to an acceptance even if, understandably, they don't like what they have to accept.

Another problem for women with breast cancer whatever their treatment is the question of 'coping'. The pressure is on all of us to appear to cope. People are praised for coping well. They are praised by hospital staff, by relatives and by friends. The apearance of coping well often belies an individual's inner state. To cope well in the short term can often mean taking much longer to confront the disease and its treatment. Part of our dignity and pride is involved in seeming to cope well in order to protect the feelings of those around us often to our own considerable cost. Continually to keep up appearances is also, while understandable, often a disservice to other women in a similar situation. If a woman with breast cancer feels she is failing because she is not 'coping', failure is added to all the other feelings. One of the great benefits of breast cancer support groups is that the feeling of *not* coping can be shared and those who have adjusted can pass on their understanding to others and also show that there is life after breast cancer.

Those who have had a mastectomy have not only to deal with their bereavement but have also to confront their sense of loss of womanhood. To regain it can not be done merely by exercise or bandages. A prosthesis can give an outward appearance of normality but it does not deal with the inner self-image. Audre Lorde, a black American woman who herself had a mastectomy, writes eloquently in the *Cancer Journals* about her struggle to confront herself following surgery but also about society's desire to patch over the surgical amputation by persuading her to wear a prosthesis so that she could go on living pretending that nothing had happened. Society too can then go on living as if nothing had happened, ignoring the thousands of women who are walking around minus one or two breasts. She argues that breast prostheses 'are offered to women after surgery in much the same way that candy is offered to babies after an injection' and that unlike other false parts given after amputation 'only false breasts are designed for appearance only, as if the only real function of women's breasts were to appear in a certain shape and size and symmetry to onlookers, or to yield to external pressure'.

Audre Lorde's attack is not on prostheses themselves nor on the women who choose to wear them but on the effect they have on attitudes to breast cancer. They conceal breast cancer and by concealing it they hinder rather than help in the struggle to find out more about its causes. They hinder the development of other forms of treatment because if you 'appear' just the same afterwards then you might as well have surgery. They compound the whole attitude to women's bodies that women's bodies are about appearance and in particular the breasts are about appearance. Finally they offer the empty comfort of 'nobody will know the difference'. But it is that very difference that Audre Lorde wishes 'to affirm, because I have lived it, and survived it, and wish to share that struggle with other women'. The important difference that she affirms is not physical but mental. It is the difference between being powerless and in a state of fear compared to the strength gained by facing death. Having done that, Audre Lorde asserts 'what is there possibly left for me to fear? Who can ever really have power over me again?'

It is the confrontation with the possibility of death that all women with breast cancer, whatever their treatment, share. There is the first shocking confrontation when diagnosis reveals a cancerous growth and then the fear grows that this time it may be the beginning of the end. For some the fear becomes a reality as different treatments successively fail to control the spread of the disease. They enter a stage where treatment becomes terminal care easing the path to death by relief of pain rather than treatment of symptoms. Women's fear that the diagnosis of breast cancer means a death sentence is not rooted in old wives' tales but rooted in hard facts. Breast cancer is the leading cause of death in this country for women between the ages of 35 and 54. The fear is also rooted in the reality of women's lives; most women know, or know of, a woman who has died from breast cancer.

Learning to confront and cope with the fear of death is hard, made harder by the fact that until recently each woman has had to do it alone. Where she is supported, loved and cared for and is able to talk about her fear then living with it can be made easier. Other women have been greatly helped by the growth of cancer self-help groups. These groups enable people with cancer or who have had cancer to share their experiences, fears, information and support. Women with breast cancer quite rightly often feel that even the most sympathetic husband, lover or friend 'does not really understand'. Cancer patients also have to deal with the attitude strongly held by many that to talk about death or the fear of death is to be morbid, and worse, by doing so, it is almost to wish it on oneself. Experience shows the reverse. Talking about death with people who do understand can help a person to confront the fear and by confronting it to be able to live with it.

Much literature on breast cancer deals with returning to life after treatment in what can best be described as a 'jolly hockey-sticks' tone. Women are advised to do their exercises, pop a prosthesis in their bra, get out and about and resume their normal life as quickly as possible and equally as quickly as possible jump into bed naked and resume sex with their husband – all literature assumes breast cancer strikes married women, not co-habitees, lesbians or single women. In some, very rare cases, it can also strike some men. The literature is clearly designed to be positive, giving women hope that normal life can be resumed. Unfortunately in its bright and breezy way it skates over the very real mental, social, sexual and physical adjustments that have to be made and to be continually re-made. Those adjustments may be made quickly, more frequently making them is a slow and painful process, sometimes they are never made. It is best to start with a recognition of the problems rather than to pretend that they are not there or that they can be dealt with easily. Recognising the problems is the first step and acting on that recognition the second. The physical problems are the easiest to deal with and those for which most help is given. The sexual problems are those which receive most public sympathy, though that does not mean that they are necessarily dealt with in private with sensitivity and sympathy. This sympathy is not however extended to women over a certain age, they are assumed, fallaciously, to have lost interest in sex and therefore not to have this problem.

Least considered have been the problems cancer creates in the mind. Not surprisingly to deal with this women have looked outside orthodox medicine for help. Self-help groups provide an increasing number with support. Alternative medicine also has a role to play following more orthodox treatment. By changing their life-style, changing their diet and by having the individual treatment provided by alternative medicine women can now get a sense of taking control of their own bodies. This can help them regain a sense of individuality after the impersonal production line of most hospital treatment. Even orthodox medical practitioners concede that mental attitudes are important to the long-term outcome. Alternative practitioners and many lay people are certain of it. But even if attitudes cannot affect the ultimate outcome they can make a substantial difference to the quality of life. That quality of life is, when life has become even more precious because it is under threat, of supreme importance.

Physical adjustments

It was another GP in the practice, who is a friend of mine, who told me about the Mastectomy Association because they sent me out of the hospital and said, 'Roll up your knickers and stuff them in your bra'.

(Jenny)

91

If you leave hospital after some form of mastectomy and without proper advice, or any advice at all, on prostheses, their availability and the range of choice, then there are people around who can help you. The Mastectomy Association was formed precisely to advise women who have had mastectomies. The service they provide is, to quote from their leaflet, 'strictly non-medical and endeavours to complement medical and nursing care by offering information about the different types of prostheses (breast forms) that are available, also bras and swimwear suitable for mastectomees, and other more personal matters'. It can take time and experimentation before a woman finds a prostheses that suits her and for her to sort out different styles of clothing. There is no doubt that women who have travelled the same road can help women who are facing the situation for the first time. Recognising this, the Mastectomy Association have a number of 'Volunteer Helpers' whom they describe as women who themselves have had mastectomies and have 'come to terms with the situation'. They are there so that 'a new mastectomee may, if she wishes, talk freely and without a time limit to someone with whom she shares a common experience – someone who has resumed her normal everyday life'. A few hospitals link up with the Mastectomy Association, allowing or even inviting voluntary helpers into the wards to talk to any patient who so wishes. For other patients they must contact the association themselves unless they have a health visitor or social worker who makes contact for them.

Women who have had a mastectomy and some women after radiotherapy have difficulty in regaining their physical mobility. Lost mobility following breast surgery is mainly caused by the removal of muscles and in particular the muscle attached to the arm. Thus getting things off shelves or reaching up can be difficult if not impossible. Before being discharged from hospital you should see a physiotherapist to be shown the exercises that you can do to regain mobility. If you are discharged without seeing a physiotherapist and find at home that you have difficulty with certain arm movements, particularly lifting the arm on the side of surgery, then ask to be referred to one at your next check-up at the hospital. It is always much easier to do exercises if they have been shown to you and also a physiotherapist can, having examined you, suggest the exercises that are best for you. Exercises can help improve mobility or even make full mobility possible again. In the absence of a physiotherapist the following exercises are a few simple ones that can help. As with all exercises you should never strain yourself. It is better to do a few and slowly build up strength. Remember it is always the arm on the side of the operation that needs the exercise.

Exercises

1. *Ball exercise.* All you need is a small soft rubber ball, a ball of wool or a piece of foam rubber. This exercise can be done from the outset lying on your back in bed with your arm raised slightly. Gently squeeze the ball several times. This will help to strengthen the hand and arm muscles.

2. *Walking up the wall.* Following a mastectomy you may well feel that metaphorically you are doing this anyway but in regaining mobility it is an exercise well worth doing in reality. To walk up the wall you need to stand barefooted facing a wall with your forehead resting against it. With your palms flat against the wall and beside your shoulders, gradually move your hands up as high as they will go. With practice you should gradually be able to move your hands higher and higher up the wall until you are able to reach right above your head with both arms straight.

3. *Hair brushing.* Raising your arm to brush your hair can present a problem, particularly getting the brush round to the back of the head. To get that mobility back practising will help. To start with, rest your elbow on a pile of books on the table or dressing table then brush your hair slowly trying to work all round. Slowly you will regain the ability to brush your hair without propping up your arm, particularly if you have been walking up the wall to regain your lifting ability.

4. *Ball on elastic.* For this exercise you need a ball with a

93

piece of elastic threaded through it. You then loop the elastic round your middle finger on the hand of your operated side. Throw the ball around in any direction and as you regain strength and mobility you will find that you will be able to catch the ball at the end of each trajectory.
5. *Bra fastening and doing up back-fastening dresses.* The action required to do both these may present problems. Practice is the best way to regain mobility until you can do both without difficulty.
6. *Breathing, posture and relaxation exercises.* Learning to walk tall again after breast surgery is not easy, not so much because of the physical problems involved in standing up straight but because of the emotional problems. Many women stoop following a mastectomy partially to reduce chest discomfort and partially as a way of trying to hide the loss of the breast. With the total healing of the scars the pain should go but the psychological scar is much harder to heal. Stooping hinders rather than helps the development of strong shoulder muscles and exercises can help you to stand straight. Other forms of help, discussed later, can make it easier for you to live with your body. Deep breathing and relaxation exercises not only help to relax your body but also your mind.

The other main physical problem following surgery is swelling in the arm (lymphœdema). This happens when lymph nodes are removed from the armpit, thus removing some of the drainage system. The fluid, unable to drain out of the arm via the lymph nodes, causes swelling. Almost all women have some swelling following surgery. This goes within a week or two but in some women the swelling never goes. With breast surgery becoming more conservative meaning the removal of less, particularly fewer surrounding muscles and lymph nodes, fewer women are suffering either extreme limitation of mobility in the affected arm or extreme swelling. But some do get swelling, which can be even more distressing and cause more long-term physical discomfort than the loss of some muscles.

Unfortunately, once swelling is there it is hard to treat. Sleeping with your arm raised above your head on a pillow helps the fluid to drain out. Suggesting it is easy, trying to get through a night with your arm in this position is not. Some women find bandaging the arm helps and it is also possible to reduce the swelling by using a mechanical device. If you are considering the latter course of action you should probably seek medical advice. One of the problems of such swelling is that it makes the arm susceptible to infection. To avoid infection try to avoid injury or cuts to the affected hand and arm. Cutting nails carefully and never cutting cuticles, wearing a thimble if sewing and wearing rubber gloves or gardening gloves when doing household or outdoor work can all help to protect the hand and arm. In general you should look after that arm with great care but if you do get a cut, a sore or cracks don't ignore them. They should be carefully washed, covered with an antiseptic cream and bandaged. Antibiotics can quickly cure any inflammation and infection but it is better to prevent them or to effect a quick cure by stopping infection developing than by having a course of antibiotics.

10. Alternative or complementary medicine

I take multi-vitamins and three iron pills a day. I've had very bad response from doctors in terms of their response to me wanting to do something. When I suggested taking vitamins they just said yes and I suggested I should take more iron because of my anaemia. The doctor said, 'It won't help the anaemia, but you can take as much iron as you like. It won't harm you to have a bit of rust.'

(Gladys)

I'm very happy with what I'm doing. I've no intention of going anywhere else: I put a letter in the magazine *Here's Health* saying how lonely it was trying to do all these things and I had a mass of letters from all over the country. People who had either had people who had died or were getting better or who'd had their lives prolonged, saying, 'You're doing the right thing because you haven't got all those side-effects to deal with. You're strengthening the immune system.'

(Jo)

For most of this century the only choice for breast cancer patients in the West was either the surgeon's knife or to do nothing. To surgery orthodox medicine has added other forms of treatment all based on cutting out or destroying the cancerous cells. This has been seen as a militaristic approach to disease. Alex Jack in the *Cancer Control Journal* (vol. 5, nos. 3/4) likens orthodox medicine's attack on cancer to the war in Vietnam. He argues,

Since the rise of the cellular hypothesis – that cancer is a mysterious, tumorous condition of localised origin – the medical establishment has sanctioned only three methods of treatment: surgery, radiation and chemotherapy. On a larger scale these are precisely the three major weapons (search-and-destroy, bombardment and chemical warfare) utilized militarily against social problems.

Alternative medicine, or as some people prefer to describe it more accurately, complementary medicine, takes a different, often slower, but more gentle approach to treating cancer. The situation now in terms of cancer treatment is one of many options. A range of choice has been opened up and into that range have entered, or re-entered, alternative and complementary forms of treatment. They have re-entered for most have their roots in ancient treatments practised for centuries both in the West and the East. Orthodox medicine and alternative medicine, a bit like sects of the Christian church, are often presented as warring sects, each fighting to discredit the other. But the patient caught up in the crossfire is not concerned with defending the beliefs of either side but with their own survival. Few patients choose to follow one camp or the other entirely. More and more they take from either side what they think will best help them. So women with breast cancer are swallowing Tamoxifen and practising what is called visualization – a method of using the power of the mind over the body. Women are having surgery and then detoxifying their body by going on the Bristol diet or are having radiotherapy and changing their diet and life-style. In their actions they question both forms of treatment, hedging their bets and taking more control of and responsibility for their own bodies.

One of the problems many women face when contemplating complementary medicine is their lack of knowledge. There is a confusing range of possibilities from healing to acupuncture and a range of practitioners from the highly skilled and responsible to quacks exploiting people's vulnerability in order to make a fast buck. Sorting through the range of alternative therapies in order to choose can be difficult and often a case of trial and error. The common element in all of them is that they all try, in varying degrees, to recruit the self-healing capacities of the body. The other common element is their treatment of the whole person, mind and body, rather than as a body without a mind, social context and individual history. This treatment of the person as a whole marks the single most significant difference between alternative approaches to cancer and orthodox approaches, for from this basic assumption stem two central beliefs that inform all types of alternative treatment. First they work on the assumption that cancer is systemic, that is, that it is in the body as a whole, and therefore chopping off bits of the body cannot get rid of it. Many believe we all have cancerous cells in us but that if our immune system is working well then they are destroyed before getting out of control. Their second basic belief is that the mind can affect the course of cancer positively or negatively. The alternative therapies for cancer therefore usually involve one or more of the following – diet, particularly using certain herbs which have a detoxifying effect on the body; homoeopathy, a system of treating like with like; acupuncture; spiritual healing and forms of psychotherapy including relaxation, meditation, visualization and various positive thinking techniques.

It is not the role of this book to detail all the different forms of complementary medicine, nor indeed do we feel qualified to evaluate them. For an introductory guide to and explanation of the range of therapies, Stephen Fulder's book *The Handbook of Complementary Medicine* is as good a starting place as any. It not only explains clearly each therapy, outlining the principles behind each approach, but it also includes addresses, further reading and lists places and standards of training. To help the lay person through the maze of alternative therapies and protect them from falling into the hands of quacks there is no doubt that a register of alternative practitioners would help. Such a system involving set standards and training will we hope soon come into being. For orthodox medicine and the State to ignore alternative medicine is to ignore the behaviour of a large number of the

British population. The Threshold Survey conducted in 1981 found that about ten million British people had consulted alternative practitioners. Ten million can hardly be all dismissed as loonies, fringe freaks and the bean brigade. To dismiss, too, other forms of medicine, such as Chinese medicine, which has been practised for as long if not much longer than Western medicine, often with good results, seems blind arrogance. One of the biggest problems for anyone contemplating alternative treatment is the cost. Only the NHS as the State-recognized form of medical treatment comes with small charges – like prescription charges, while others not recognized have to be paid for. Charges vary enormously, many practitioners charging according to the person's ability to pay. But the mere fact of having to pay puts them out of reach of a large number of people in Britain. The treatments cost money too. Changing diet can be costly, although for those on supplementary benefit it is possible to claim an additional allowance for special diets required for illness. However such a diet will not always be accepted, particularly if it is not sanctioned by an orthodox practitioner. Most of the diets are based on organically grown food and on vitamin supplements, both hard to get and expensive. Vitamins clearly do have an important role to play, but a word of warning: some vitamins like B6 taken in large quantities can be toxic and it is wise therefore not to do so without taking advice. Many people also find the radical dietary change is not just expensive and time consuming, but anti-social and isolating as well. It isolates the individual from other people, particularly around the meal table. Many women with breast cancer often have families and prefer to make small changes to the general dietary habits of their family as a whole than to eat a separate diet.

Some alternative therapies are based on a critique of con-temporary Western ways of life, the argument being that our life-styles are contributory to the diseases we get, particularly cancer. Besides diet (what we eat and drink) stress is rated high in causing disease. Because of this many therapies are based on encouraging patients to change their life-styles. This is easy to suggest but often fails to take into account the realities of most people's lives. Life is stressful, caught up as we are in the struggle to earn money or to live on the dole, or to live in what is often an inhuman environment of tower blocks or de-personalized estates and to bring up children with little support. It is not easy for the majority to change their life-style, and for some the surgeon's knife may well seem an easier, less stressful option than seeking alternative therapies and the cash to pay for them.

There is a further problem. To question someone's life-style, valid as it may be in trying to treat a disease, the danger is run of inculcating the patient with guilt: guilt that they have, through the life that they have led, caused their own disease. Guilt is the last thing a cancer patient needs or ought to feel. Women already carry around with them too great a burden of guilt and no treatment should increase that burden. Instead it should help them to unyoke themselves of that guilt. Our lives *are* stressful and there is no doubt that being able to lead less stressful lives would make us happier and healthier. To suggest that we are capable of such change is often further to burden us. For most of us, such change can only come about through fundamental economic, social and political change. Meditating may make us calmer but it can't pay the rent; self-analysis can change the way we see ourselves but may not necessarily change the relationships around us; acupuncture may heal our bodies but it can't provide a job, let alone a satisfying one. This comment is not to say that meditation, self-analysis and acupuncture aren't, in their different ways, of help, but that broader social change is required to create a different, less stressful world with a changed value system for us all.

In a patronising way orthodox practitioners will concede that alternative therapies help by making the patient think more positively. The following from *Cancer* by Smedley, Sikora and Stepney sums up the orthodox attitude:

> The fairest conclusion is that the various alternative
> approaches may be helpful in supporting cancer patients
> and their relatives. Self-help, and the idea that the patient

should develop a positive attitude to the disease, and not simply become a passive recipient of a complex factory-like treatment programme, are beneficial. But there is no basis for making wildly optimistic claims that these treatments bring about a cure.

It is true that alternative treatments of breast cancer are not proven while the orthodox treatments may be statistically measured. That measurement, however, hardly produces figures to be boasted about. Clearly more evidence about alternative therapies would be welcomed as a means of evaluating them, but to judge the one form of medicine against the other on survival statistics alone is to misunderstand the difference between the two approaches. While both are concerned with saving life, alternative medicine is equally concerned with its quality for however long there is life. The fact that people go to alternative medicine to be treated as people and that alternative therapies give the individual the sense that they can take responsibility for their lives is of profound importance. Jo Spence, a woman with breast cancer who after primary orthodox treatment chose alternative therapies, writes of the different effect on the individual that each form of treatment has. Of orthodox medicine she comments:

> Whilst not wishing to deny the care and dedication of most National Health Service personnel, the patient is routinely infantilized, and placed in a position of total powerlessness whilst surrogate mummies and daddies (doctors and nurses) carry out their prescribed hierarchical tasks.

In contrast, in alternative therapies,

> The patient is encouraged to take some responsibility for getting and staying better. At worst, this means more work for the patient and an ability to make informed decisions. At best, it means a complete change of lifelong habits in relation to food, drugs, exercise, and the awakening

knowledge that the body can not deal forever with a
completely unharmonious relationship with one's psychic,
social, living and working environment.

(New Socialist, October 1985)

Jo Spence recognized that alternative therapies (she finally
opted for Chinese medicine) did not promise her a cure, but did
give her a new perspective on her own life and on the need to
'understand the politics woven into the deepest levels of our
personal lives'.

Many women are taking more responsibility for their own
well-being. If a doctor ignores their questions about vitamins,
diet change or the benefit of relaxation they are increasingly
going elsewhere to have those questions answered. Patients are
voting with their feet in questioning orthodox treatments and
attitudes. Equally, most, apart from a few zealous converts,
approach alternative therapies with a questioning mind. The
assumption that people who go to alternative therapies are either
cranks or those for whom all else has failed is untrue. There are
some for whom alternative therapies are a last desperate
measure, but for most they are a way of taking some responsibility
for their lives. *Complementary* medicine is the more apt term for
the reality of the situation. Almost all the women we talked to
who have or have had breast cancer mixed orthodox and
complementary medicine, taking something from each and thus
exercising their right of choice. It is clear that behind that choice
is a determination by women to beat the disease rather than to be
beaten by it. They don't want to be statistics but individuals who
can prove there is life, and a life of quality, after breast cancer.

11. Why me – why us?

I would say the significant thing, in my family, is that
almost all the women on my father's side have had breast
cancer. They were all encouraged to read medicine or
become missionaries and did their bit preaching to the
unconverted in the jungle and then married out there in
their late twenties – a responsible age. One aunt was a
colonel in the army. I think she was about 38 when she
married. And the only one who hasn't had breast cancer is
my elder sister and she is now 51. She was married young.
We all thought she was too young when she went down the
aisle. She loved her chap, and off she went and had two
children very young.

(Jenny)

I came from a family that was probably very repressed – an
awful lot of church teaching, etc. Sometimes I wonder
whether with breast cancer it's not so much the people who
have babies late but the people who have sex late, and who
therefore have long years of repression.

(Hazel)

Every woman who gets breast cancer asks herself, 'Why me?'
and that inevitably leads to questions about one's individual life
and what elements in it might have triggered a cancerous
tumour. Some find no answers, some are sure of their own
personal cause and others look to the bad luck of their genes. It is
impossible to say with any certainty, except of the Japanese
women exposed to radiation from the atomic bomb, why any one

103

individual gets breast cancer. It is equally impossible to say with any certainty why, in Britain, one woman in twelve gets breast cancer, or why that incidence is, worryingly, on the increase. So far no one cause had been isolated, nor indeed have a number of definite causes been found. There are, however, many speculative assertions about the probable causes, some of which are based on more evidence than others.

Many studies have been conducted to try to find the causes of breast cancer and from all these carried out so far, both in Britain and elsewhere, only two clear findings emerge. They relate to women in high-risk groups and to women in low-risk groups. Those most at risk have a history of breast cancer in the family. If your mother, sister, grandmother or daughter have had breast cancer then your risk is greater, in fact it almost doubles. Women in this high-risk group should always be vigilant and examine themselves regularly. They should also raise the question of regular screening with their doctor. Women in this group may also wish to think about changing their diet, as a preventive measure (see below). They might also think of exploring alternative preventive therapies that include other measures besides dietary changes. Low-risk women are those who started menstruating late and who have their first child before the age of 25.

Because the incidence of breast cancer varies greatly from country to country much research has been focused on the different life-styles of different groups of women. Research has looked at why women in such countries as Mexico, China and Japan have a significantly lower incidence of breast cancer than women in Britain, USA, Denmark and Israel. One of the earliest areas of research was to study whether breast-feeding had any bearing on the subsequent development of breast cancer. No correlation was found, but the belief that there is one still lingers on in the minds of many women although researchers have long since dismissed it.

There was, at one time, considerable concern about the potentially cancer-forming long-term effect of the drug used (Stilbestrol) quite freely and liberally in Britain to dry up women's milk supply. The recent increase in breast cancer in Britain may well be partly due to the widespread use of it for a period of time. Concern about the possible carcinogenic potential of the drug led to its withdrawal. Letting milk-filled breasts dry up naturally may be more painful, but it is infinitely safer than drug-induced drying up.

Another slightly more profitable area of research has been into dietary factors. This research was inspired by studies which revealed that Japanese women, apart from those exposed to radiation following the atomic bombs on Hiroshima and Nagasaki, have a low incidence of breast cancer. That incidence, however, increased when Japanese women moved to live in North America, until through successive generations the incidence in Japanese Americans equals those of other American women. Diet was found to be one of the biggest differences between their Japanese way of life and their new American life. In particular the move from Japan to America was a move from a low-fat to high-fat diet. Subsequent research has shown some correlation between high-fat diets and the incidence of breast cancer. People on high-fat diets have higher proportions of certain bacteria in their bowels. These bacteria are able to produce oestrogens and it is known that such oestrogens are potentially cancer-causing in the breast. Besides a high fat intake in general being regarded as possibly cancer-causing, milk and milk products in particular are under question. Western countries are the countries with the highest incidence of breast cancer and are the countries in which dairy produce forms a considerable part of the diet. Most people in Asia, Africa and China after weaning lose the enzyme lactase which is necessary for lactose (milk sugar) to be broken down, absorbed and digested, because they are not fed dairy products. Most adults outside the West are incapable of digesting lactose. As yet no direct link between dairy products and breast cancer has been found, but dairy products must, until proven innocent, be under suspicion.

Diet is by no means the only difference in the life-styles of women on different continents. Patterns of development and child-bearing also differ greatly and they have been the subject of studies. One of the significant differences between poor and rich countries is the age at which girls start menstruating. Western girls start on average considerably earlier than girls in the Third World. Studies have found a correlation between the age of menstruation and breast cancer; the later a woman starts the less the risk. It is not known, though, whether it is the age of onset of menstruation that is important or the number of menstrual cycles before the first pregnancy. Many Third World women start menstruating late, conceive their first child after only a few cycles and have a very low incidence of breast cancer. The large number of menstrual cycles in Western women between the start of menstruation and late first pregnancy is by no means proven as a reason for the higher incidence of breast cancer, but there is enough evidence to warrant further study. However, such studies have to be evaluated cautiously. The fact that the first line of research into the causes of breast cancer was based on trying to ascertain whether breast-feeding reduced the risk of breast cancer, and indeed many women still wrongly believe it does, cannot help but make one suspicious of all lines of research directed to trying to reaffirm women's role as 'naturally' that of breeders and feeders. There are those like Drs Andrew and Penny Stanway, authors of *The Breast*, who clearly believe that women's emancipation has brought upon them a range of diseases including breast cancer. Their solution to the 'current situation with women's reproductive ills' is that 'with the probable decreasing need for people to work over the next few decades perhaps we shall see a return to more biological mothering, earlier child-bearing and, who knows, even a return to a more stable family life as a result'. In other words women's health, the family's health and the nation's health is dependant on women getting back to child-bearing as early and as often as possible. What they fail to take into account is all the other mental and physical diseases suffered by women caused precisely by their role as child-bearers, child-rearers and holders of the family together.

Central to research into breast cancer has been the study of hormones, those our body produce and those we put into our body in the form of the contraceptive pill, in hormone replacement therapy for menopausal women (HRT) and through a high-fat diet. One of the problems in trying to evaluate the results of research into the effect of hormones is that behind much of it lie vested interests, particularly those of the rich and powerful drug companies. Research is rarely 'pure'. Just as some researchers hope that their findings will confirm their belief that women would be healthier (and society happier) if they reverted to their role of full-time child-bearers, so, too, do the drug companies, paying for much research, hope to prove that there is no correlation between the contraceptive pill and breast cancer. The results of research into a possible relationship between breast cancer and taking the contraceptive pill are in some areas contradictory. Two recent studies done in the USA and in New Zealand confirmed earlier surveys that women who had taken the pill even for as long as 15 years ran no increased risk of getting breast cancer. This was questioned by Swedish researchers who in 1986 reported that they had found that women who had taken the pill for 12 years or longer did run an increased risk and there was a question mark about those who had taken it for more than 8 years. Given the confusion, women who take the contraceptive pill can best protect themselves by ensuring it is a low dose one and they should consider not taking it for more than 8 years. Those who have taken the pill for more than eight years should discuss with their doctor being screened regularly. All research to date seems agreed that taking the pill for only a few years does not increase the risk of getting breast cancer and indeed it can reduce the risk of benign, non-concerous breast disorders. There is concern, however, about hormone replacement therapy. Studies have found that women taking hormones in this form actually run a slightly increased risk.

Many other studies are also being conducted into the causes of breast cancer. One line of study is looking into the possibility that a virus which can be transmitted through breast-feeding from mother to daughter is the cause. Experiments with mice have shown that if their milk contains a virus called the Bitner virus, it can be passed on to their offspring and it is known to be potentially cancer-causing (carcinogenic). A study of a small group of Iranian women living in an isolated community who have a one in five chance of developing breast cancer found that their milk contained viral particles similar to the Bitner virus, but these findings have not been followed up elsewhere, leaving the question still unanswered. Ionizing radiation is know to increase the risk of breast cancer. Japanese women exposed to radiation from the atomic bombs at Hiroshima and Nagasaki have shown a high incidence; the greater their exposure the higher the risk. Knowing that, the question then is what level of exposure to radiation can cause breast cancer. There is considerable debate about it and we will discuss it in more detail in the following section on screening.

The other main line of research has been, as with other forms of cancer, into the degree to which stress can be cancer causing. One study found a higher incidence of breast cancer in women who had experienced a major traumatic event, such as bereavement, than in those who had not. There are those, too, who believe that certain personalities, those prone to depression, stress and introversion, are more likely to develop the disease. There is a growing body of evidence that stress is related to the development of cancer, but it is hard to measure stress or the ways in which people cope with it. For the ways of coping are probably as important as the stress itself.

There is no answer to the question 'Why me?' and as yet there is no answer to the question British women could put to themselves, 'Why us?' The latter does seem to be the more pertinent question, though each woman, faced with the reality of her own disease, is bound to question her own bad fortune. In order to halt the rise in the incidence of breast cancer and better still to bring it down, the question 'Why us?' must be asked. Something about us, our life-style, our environment, our genes, causes a rate of breast cancer in us nearly five times higher than among women of other continents. In answering the question, many women's lives could be saved and many others kept from the trauma and distress of breast cancer and its treatment.

While large sums of money are spent on research into different forms of treatment for breast cancer and into developing new drugs, more sophisticated forms of radiotherapy and better implants, very little money is spent on research into why so many British women develop it in the first place. The National Health Service does not exist to make profits, but the drug companies, manufacturers of medical equipment, prostheses and implants all do and some of the profits from breast cancer and the orthodox forms of treatment are very large. There is little profit to be made by any manufacturer in finding the cause of breast cancer unless that cause can be treated with one of their products. If the government was seriously interested in prevention rather than treatment then it would invest in research into causes, but the sums it makes available for such research are small.

Those with breast cancer will ask 'Why me?', but those women who have not developed it should take on the responsibility of asking 'Why us?'. We should ask it for our own self-protection and for the protection of our daughters, granddaughters, mothers and women friends.

12. Breast self-examination and screening

> I still think I'm going to examine myself every month
> because that lump could have been a sign that I'm going to
> get it. But they never told me anything even how to
> examine my breasts when I came out.
>
> (Ann)

In all the debates about breast cancer one fact is generally agreed: early detection gives the patient a much greater chance of survival. The rate of survival beyond five years goes up to between 80 and 90 per cent if the lump is small- marble-sized or smaller- when first treated and if there is no evidence of spread. Dr Albert Milan, an American who has written a whole book on the need for and technique of breast self-examination, claims that 'Failure to detect breast cancer in its earliest stages is the single greatest redeemable sin in the entire cancer confrontation.'

While research into the cause of breast cancer could be the other great 'redeemable sin' in the reduction of the incidence of breast cancer, there is no doubt that early detection is the route to reducing the number of deaths in those who get it. The two main methods available are self-examination and screening by X-ray. It is around the latter method, mammography, that debate has raged – to screen or not to screen, the costs, the benefits and the risks. There has been little doubt about the benefit of examining one's own breasts. Most lumps are already found by women themselves or by their partners. Breast self-examination is designed to encourage women to find lumps through examination and not by accident. It is a first important step for women in taking responsibility for the well-being and future of their own bodies. It is a safe method that costs nothing except a little time each month. Although the very earliest and smallest growths cannot be detected by this means, a woman who knows the look and feel of her own breasts can often feel a lump even smaller than a marble.

If breast self-examination can, in most cases, make the difference between just a few years of life and the prospect of living out a 'natural' life, why do so many women not examine themselves? The reason appears to lie in the lack of education about how we can take responsibility for our own bodies and in the fact that so many women feel alienated from their bodies. Another reason is simply fear of what they might find. Health education has been sadly lacking from the curricula of schools. We think of health as something looked after by doctors, despite the fact that most children know the rhyme 'An apple a day keeps the doctor away'. Few parents or teachers have translated the message of that rhyme into the recognition that preventive medicine can help to keep you healthy. Nor have they made it into a serious subject for study. Most children leave school having learned almost nothing about the way that their bodies function, let alone about how to care for them. A good education should include that knowledge, and girls should be taught not only how their reproductive system works but what can go wrong with it. Learning how to examine one's own breasts should be included in education for self-care and girls should be encouraged to start doing it routinely and regularly so that it is an established part of their life before they enter the real 'danger years' after the age of 35. As important as learning to examine their breasts is learning to confront their own bodies. Most of the women we talked to knew about self-examination but hadn't practised it. They said that they didn't like the idea of doing it or that they didn't do it for fear of what they might find. Learning to do it cannot take away the fear, but it can take away the deep resistance many women have to feeling their own bodies.

Seeing women's bodies as sexual objects encourages this resistance; as objects most women do not like their bodies very much. They are uneasy with their shape, size or skin texture.

Few can look in the mirror and accept the image they see without wishing that in some way they were different. Breasts in particular are objects: objects for other people to look at or feel; objects that are a source of sexual pleasure both privately and, more so, publicly in their daily display in newspapers and elsewhere. Only in private and rarely in public is it acknowledged that breasts are for breast-feeding. Men gazing at page 3 models don't want to know that inside those two objects of sexual titillation are a whole network of lobules, ductiles and ducts designed for producing milk. But it is that complex milk production system that makes them so prone to disorders. Women should be able or should be taught to see and feel their own breasts and be at ease doing so. It is not dirty groping but healthy examination. It is a crazy world where women are so 'created' for men that they find it acceptable for a man to touch their breasts, but not themselves.

The fear of self-examination can only be countered by publicising the fact that the earlier breast cancer is detected the greater the chance of long-term survival and the greater the chance surgeons will suggest removing the lump only and not the whole breast. Early detection can be life saving and breast saving. That message should be engraved in women's minds. Women should remember it whenever they recoil from examining their own breasts or when they think they won't bother to do it for a month, or two or three. GPs, practitioners at Well Woman clinics and those in hospitals could and should play a much more active role in encouraging breast self-examination. Women are not taught how to do it. Even those who have had a 'scare' are sent home from a breast clinic without having it and the reasons for it explained. Most Well Woman clinics examine women's breasts as part of their programme but their attempts to teach women rarely go further than putting up a poster on the wall showing how it should be done. If you are not sure how to do it, or whether you are doing it right, ask someone experienced to show you.

In the absence of anyone having taught you – here is a step-by-step guide:

When, where and how often

Breast self-examination should be done regularly once a month. Pre-menopausal women should do it just after their period has finished because this is the time when the breasts, because of their monthly cycle, have the least additional fluid in them. Post-menopausal women need to allocate one day a month which is inscribed in their memory or in their diary. Choosing the first day of the month is at least memorable. Regularity is important for it is through regular self-examination that any change can be seen or felt. It also takes a few months to learn what one's own breasts really feel and look like. All breasts feel and look different, and they change with the years.

The examination shouldn't take much more than 10 minutes. If you have a shower, part of it can be done there. For the rest of the examination you need to be somewhere where you are relaxed, warm, have a good mirror and a place you can lie down. Most women also prefer to do it in private.

Looking

1. Strip to the waist and stand in front of a mirror with your arms hanging relaxed by your sides. Have a good look at your breasts to get a clear image of them. Look to see whether one is larger than the other, one higher than the other and whether the nipples are similar in size and position. Turn slightly from side to side, again studying your breasts. You will repeat this every month so it is important to get a clear image of them so that you can notice any change (see Diagram 3).
2. Put your hands on the crown of your head. Look in the mirror, turning from side to side.
3. With your arms still up put the palms of your hands together just in front of your forehead and squeeze the palms tightly together and then release them. This contracts and releases the muscles on which the breasts are situated. Do this facing the mirror and look while you are turning from side to side.

Diagram 3 Looking

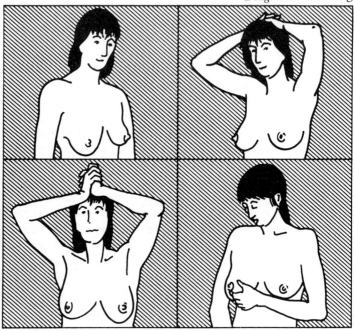

All three methods are designed to show you whether there is any evidence of a change in the size or shape of either breast, any change in the nipple axis, that is, one pulling upwards or outwards, any sign of the breast bulging, indenting, retracting, dimpling or any change in the skin surface, particularly if the skin looks in any way like orange peel.

4. Finally, look at your nipples and the area of brown skin around them. You need to inspect them for any sign of ulcers, eczema, sebaceous cysts or other skin conditions. Look carefully to see if they show any sign of change as though they are, or one is, flattening, inverting or dimpling. If you have noticed any discharge from either nipple try gently to express some of it. This you do by gently stroking the nipple with your thumb and forefinger starting from about an inch away from the nipple and stroking inwards to it. If any discharge appears, note what colour it is, whether it is bloody or not and whether it comes

from two nipples or one, and if just one nipple, whether it seems to come from just one duct.

Feeling

1. The shower or the bath are good places in which to examine your breasts. Both are warm, relaxing places where you feel your body anyway while washing it. Always use the hand opposite the breast you are feeling, so you use the right hand to examine the left breast and vice versa. However, women with large breasts if examining them standing up may need to use both hands one for support while the other is feeling (see Diagram 4).

Diagram 4 Feeling

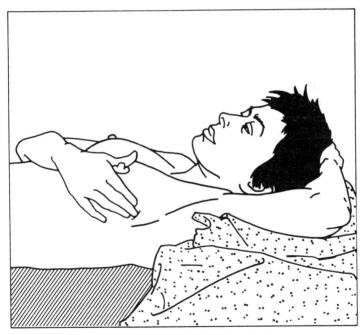

Using the opposite hand with the fingers held together, press gently around the nipple area and then slowly work round the breast in circles moving outwards until you have felt the whole

115

breast. The number of circles will depend on the size of your breast. Feel too the area above and around your breast and particularly under the arm. As a double check, raise each arm and while it is raised repeat the process of feeling the breast, the under arm and the area above the breast. Always use the hand on the opposite side from the breast you are examining.

2. Next lie down on a bed, a couch or on the floor; wherever you feel comfortable and most at ease will do. Put a small pillow or rolled-up towel under the shoulder of the side you are to examine. Place the arm on the side you are to examine up and over the forehead. As with the procedure used in the bath or shower, with the flat ends of your fingers held together feel round the nipple working outwards in circles until the whole breast has been felt and then feel under the arm and the area around the breast. Do this twice. First with your other arm resting on your forehead, and then with it beside your body. Use both methods again to examine the other breast.

What you are feeling for is anything like a lump or change in the tissues of the breasts and in the area under the arm. It takes some time to get used to the feel of your breasts but once you have done so you will be able to detect any change or growth.

If you think that there is any change in the look or feel of your breasts, in the area around them, in particular under the arm, or in either of your nipples, then you should go and have it checked out. Remember, early detection could be life and breast saving.

Most women do detect their own lumps, some detect them quite early but many detected lumps go unreported. Some women wait weeks, months and sometimes years before going to see anyone about them. Some women hope that they will go away, some are paralysed with fear and a few are ignorant of the possible implications. Most are plain frightened, frightened of cancer and of losing a breast. The medical profession could do much to help with this problem. If their approach to breast cancer was more sympathetic and understanding and was backed up by more open minds about different forms of treatment, many women would be less terrified of reporting their lumps. They would not feel that a lump meant the immediate end of them as women as a result of mastectomy and a fairly immediate death from cancer. Women themselves can help by making public their experiences of breast cancer and the fact that many live on, some without a breast and some having managed to conserve their breasts. Women can help to modify the terror felt by other women.

Screening

The other main form of early detection is through screening by some form of image gathering. Various ways of getting an image of the inside of the breast have been tried. Thermography is one way. It is a relatively safe diagnostic method based on the fact that cancerous growths radiate more heat than healthy tissue. An infra-red picture of the breast is gathered; cancerous cells, the hot spots, showing up as dark spots. Though, safe, unfortunately thermography has so far not proved to be very reliable. It fails to pick up quite a high percentage of detectable growths. Another method is called ultrasonography. It is better known to women who have been or are pregnant. The image is made by bouncing sound frequencies off internal organs which are then by a computer, translated into a screen image which a diagnostician can read. Unfortunately, like thermography, it has so far produced unreliable results in detecting breast cancer. There is hope that with time and research one of these two methods may be refined so that they do give reliable results.

There is a comparatively new and extremely expensive way of trying to detect cancerous growths based on radio frequency signals. This form of scanning is called nuclear magnetic resonance. The patient is placed in a magnetic field and is scanned by radio pulses which stimulate signals in the atoms of the body. Cancer cells emit signals with different radio frequencies from healthy cells. These signals are received and turned into an image on a screen. As far as it is known it is both a safe and an effective means of gathering information about cancerous cells, but it is extremely costly. Few hospitals in Britain have been able to afford the half million pounds or so that a nuclear magnetic resonance scanner costs. So far then the only form of image gathering that is not too astronomically expensive and that produces results that have a high degree of accuracy is mammography. Unfortunately the safety of mammography has been questioned.

Mammography is a form of X-ray using radiation. At least two images from different angles are needed to build up a picture of each breast and from them to be able to detect any sign of cancerous growth. While few question the use of mammography once and the small exposure to radiation that one X-ray causes, much doubt has been expressed about the cumulative effect of the repeated X-ray doses that regular screening would incur. The defenders of mammography claim that the levels of radiation in modern low-dose mammography are so small that they cannot put the patient at risk. Those opposing that view believe that any level of radiation is dangerous in that radiation is known to cause cancer. Questioning the use of mammography in screening, the journal of the American Medical Association wrote in February 1977:

> High risk of breast cancer is said to the associated with genetic factors, pre-existing benign breast disease, artificial menopause, family history of breast cancer, failure to breast-feed, older age at time of first pregnancy, high socioeconomic status, specific blood groups, fatty diet, obesity and hormonal imbalances. But none of these factors is as certain a cause of cancer in the breast as is radiation.

It is hard at this point to judge which group has right on their side. Until a group of women have been screened over a long period and the long-term effects are measured there is no way of judging. But its opponents would argue that no group of women should ever be subject to the risk of such a trial. There are those, too who believe in alternative medicine and who not only question mammography and the dangers of exposure to radiation but also the benefit of detecting very early cancerous growths. Brenda Kidman in *A Gentle Way With Cancer* writes, objecting to all forms of early detection, that

> Microscopic tumours probably come and go due to the efficiency of the body's natural defence system. The only positive benefit from an early warning device would be to alert the individual to the fact that it was time to start doing something positive about a life-style which was obviously undermining his or her own health.

For those who wish for early detection, mammography does have that facility. Various trials have been conducted into the benefit of regular screening by mammography and are being conducted in Britain at this moment. Dr Barbara Thomas of the Guildford Breast Cancer Screening Unit believes screening can reduce mortality from breast cancer. It can do so because mammography can pick up very small tumours and all the evidence shows that small tumours treated very quickly with no evidence of lymph node involvement have a very good prognosis. At least 80 per cent of women in that category survive for at least 10 years after primary treatment; the study has not been done for long enough to give overall long-term survival rates. One of the big criticisms of mammography has been whether the not insubstantial cost of regularly screening women would be of benefit to women in leading to a reduction of mortality. Ideally, of course, cost should not be considered, but for governments funding the health service and for those administrators in the health service deciding where their increasingly scant resources should be put, cost and benefit are prime considerations. While cuts in the costs of the machinery required for mammography are unlikely unless companies are compelled by government to reduce their profits, Dr Barbara Thomas does have views on how the costs of a screening programme could be cut. She sees no reason why properly trained nurses with experience could not run screening centres, thus cutting out the need for doctors on high salaries.

The most recent trial conducted into the benefits of screening by mammography was conducted in Sweden and the results were reported in 1985. They broadly confirmed both the findings from a trial in New York, which were reported in the early 1970s, and research done in Holland. The Swedish trial was aimed at finding out whether it is possible to prevent women from dying from breast cancer by early detection. The trial involved 160,000 women half of whom were screened at two-year intervals by mammography and the other half, the control group, were not. A discussion of the ethics of such trials is not our concern in this section (see section on trial areas), although the use of control groups has to be questioned. The use of a control group needs further questioning in the light of the results. They found one-third fewer deaths from breast cancer in the screened group than in the control group. This lowering of mortality rates was almost certainly a result of the early detection of small tumours. The benefit though was found to be for women in the 50 to 74 age group. The screened women in the age group 40 to 50 showed no appreciable benefit from having been screened over the control group. The reasons for this are possibly to be found in the fact that mammography is less accurate in picking up cancerous growths in the breasts of pre-menopausal women and that younger women tend to have faster-growing cancers and therefore screening every two years is not frequent enough. The overall finding of the trial was that regular screening can lead to a reduction of deaths from breast cancer in women over the age of 50.

A similar trial in Britain has confirmed the Swedish findings that screening of women over the age of 50 can detect very small cancerous lumps and can save lives. Over 15,000 women die from breast cancer every year in Britain and it is estimated that a nationwide screening service for women between the ages of 50 and 64 could save at least 4,000 women's lives a year. Responding to the research findings and to pressure from women, the Conservative Government announced in early 1987 its intention of committing money to enable a nationwide screening service for women between 50 and 64 to be established. Training sufficient people to do the mammograms and to interpret the x-rays inevitably will take time, however it is estimated that given the limited amount of money the Government is prepared to commit it will take at least ten years before the service is operational. Such a commitment is an important start but women will have to keep up the pressure to ensure that the Government's policy is made practice and does not go into the annals of history as merely a vote-getting policy. In the wake of the scandal about the lack of system in and inefficiencies of the cervical screening programme there can be little immediate optimism that the more expensive screening of women for breast cancer will be quickly, systematically and efficiently introduced.

Until there is a nationwide screening programme women over the age of 50 can ask to be screened. Demand creates supply and by doing so each individual woman can protect herself and be lobbying for the service. Women in the high risk categories should also demand to be screened. For the rest, breast self-examination is a safe and reasonably effective method of detecting cancerous growths. Women of whatever age, and whether they are being screened or not, can be their own early-detector system by making breast self-examination a regular event in their lives.

13. Women's experiences

The case histories given below have not been selected because they are typical or untypical. We did not set out to talk to any group of women who either had one particular form of treatment or who held one set of attitudes. Because we, the authors, both live in London and could not afford to travel far, almost all those whose experiences are included live in the south-east. The fact that they are based on women prepared to talk of their experiences and feelings also means that excluded are those women who are unable to confront their disease and talk about it. Sadly there are many women with breast cancer who are invisible except as statistics.

Most of the following case histories are based on interviews which, because they often took several hours and frequently diverted from the main subject, have had to be edited down. Although each case history is clearly the experience of one individual many common themes emerge. It is those common themes that we have tried to address in the rest of the book; here women talk for themselves of their own experiences.

Jill

Jill was 37 when she discovered a lump in her breast. She refused a mastectomy and agreed only to the surgical removal of the lump. Surgery was followed by a prophylactic course of chemotherapy and a course of radiotherapy. Five years after her first treatment Jill discovered a lump in the same breast. Following a biopsy confirming that it was a cancerous recurrence she started hormone therapy – Tamoxifen. Her son was born after having had several miscarriages when she was 35.

I was getting dressed one morning and I caught sight of my breast in the mirror and saw a dimple. I lay on the bed and felt it. That afternoon I went to see the GP and she confirmed that there was a lump and referred me to the breast clinic at the local hospital.

I had a mammogram and a needle biopsy and immediately after the biopsy the surgeon assured me he thought the lump was innocent. It was only a week later, on Good Friday, during the lengthy wait to have the stitches removed, that I began to suspect that something was wrong. For having been a nurse for 20 years and knowing how the hospital system works, all their attempts to reassure me that the delay was only caused by the time it was taking 'to get a trolley ready' didn't convince me. Eventually he arrived and as we were going into a cubicle I said to him 'I know what you want to see me for'. I can still see his face – he looked absolutely shocked. 'Oh yes, you used to be a nurse,' he replied and added, as we were still going to the cubicle, 'Yes it is bad news.' He was as blunt as that. He then removed the stitches and whilst he was doing so told me that I could be readmitted on Easter Monday for a mastectomy on Tuesday. I was assured it was very simple surgery and that I would be home on the following Friday.

I felt numb – shocked – and I heard myself say, 'No, no mastectomy.' The argument then began. Most of what he said was emotional blackmail, the gist of which was 'Don't worry about yourself. Your responsibility is to your husband and your children.' In the course of the argument I asked that further tests should be done, in particular, a liver and bone scan to see if there was any spread of the disease. He agreed on the condition that I would see the consultant surgeon after the tests. Then he insisted on seeing my husband and tried to persuade him that mastectomy was the only answer. My husband disagreed with him, supporting me and my decision.

I got home and cried and kept crying from Friday to

Monday night. My GP gave me some Valium and
Mogadon which I took but it didn't help. On Monday
evening I felt filled with self-disgust; I can't tell you how I
looked. My eyes were so swollen I couldn't close them or
open them properly. At least my self-disgust motivated me
to have a constructive discussion with my husband, for
initially neither of us had been able to talk about it. Out of
that discussion came my resolve to use my privilege as an
ex-nurse to find out through contacts I had in the medical
profession as much as I could about breast cancer and
different treatments. What I found out confirmed my
resolve not to have a mastectomy.

After the bone and liver scan, which were both negative,
I saw the consultant surgeon. He, like his colleague,
insisted that mastectomy was the only answer for me and
that if I continued to refuse surgery then I would be
responsible for my own imminent death. He gave me a life
expectancy of two years (that was six years ago) and made
the general comment that 'it's a shame women are learning
more about their bodies as it's making my job more
difficult'. The other thing he said which appalled me was,
'I understand you know some radiotherapist somewhere
and that he had advised you. *I* deal with breast cancer all
the time.' I had consulted my radiotherapist friend
precisely because he treats cancer full-time whereas I know
the consultant was a general surgeon. It was clear that
further discussion with the consultant was useless and so I
requested to be referred to a woman at another London
hospital which my consumer research had led me to believe
would offer an alternative treatment to mastectomy. That
was done without delay.

I saw Dr X a few days later. The difference in attitude
was incredible, in spite of the fact that a referral letter had
preceeded me describing me as 'difficult and emotional'. At
that first appointment we discussed my case at length and a
whole range of alternative treatments and probable
consequences. She offered me a choice of reconsidering

mastectomy or of having a course of radiotherapy followed by a course of chemotherapy. In offering the latter treatment she explained to me such a course of treatment would be long and fairly harrowing. I chose the latter course, and it was long and harrowing.

The course of radiotherapy consisted of daily treatments for three months with weekends off. The side effects were unpleasant, mainly acute fatigue and acute discomfort from the effects of radiotherapy on the treated skin. When the course of radiotherapy was finished I had a month off and we all went, as a family, on holiday. On return from our holiday I started the course of chemotherapy. At three-weekly intervals I had to have eight injections of a 'cocktail' of anti-cancer drugs. They were given to me as an insurance policy against the spread of rogue cells. The side effects were not as bad as I expected them to be. After each injection I suffered 24 hours of nausea and the culminative effect of the drugs caused some temporary thinning of the hair.

Throughout the treatment, of course I had moments of doubt. In fact my worst moments of doubt were during the year following the treatment, especially as the consultant had given me a life expectancy of two years. Whilst I had been declared cancer-free, my confidence in living three score years and ten had been destroyed.

Unfortunately five years after the original lump a new lump appeared where the first one had been. It was August and only two months after my last check-up when all had seemed fine. After finding the new lump I ignored it for about two weeks, trying to explain it to myself as part of the radiation damage my breast had had. Eventually I asked my husband to feel it and he agreed it was a new lump. I went straight back to the hospital and my doctor, a radiotherapist, also thought it was suspect. She immediately got an opinion from the surgeon who thought the same. Once again a mastectomy was suggested – this time with the bonus of an implant to follow. I still resisted.

125

I only consented to have a biopsy done under local anaesthetic. I wanted to be sure that they did not cut out any more than strictly necessary. The biopsy was extremely quick and pretty painful but I was able to leave the hospital 20 minutes after coming out of the theatre. My husband and I went and had a lovely Indian meal.

A week after the biopsy I got the results which confirmed all our suspicions. My doctor immediately put me on Tamoxifen. After a month taking it there was a dramatic reduction in the size of the lump and it has continued to get smaller. They say Tamoxifen has very few side-effects but I am sure it has given me headaches, accentuated my depression and has stopped my periods. The worst physical thing at the moment is the hole I have where the biopsy was done. When the three stitches were removed after the biopsy the scar opened and now six months later I still have a deep hole about the size of a walnut. It's unpleasant, distressing and a constant reminder of the illness. My GP referred me to the Homoeopathic Hospital for treatment to try to heal the hole. After a short period of treatment it is beginning to get smaller.

I've been much more devastated this time round. I've had times of real despair and long periods of depression. To be struck again when you think you've just passed the five-year survival period seems very cruel. It's difficult for my husband and my children and this time the children are old enough to have some understanding. They find the hole distressing to see and the family and friends have to live with my irrational behaviour. This time, although it was a bigger blow, I've had much more help and support. I'm particularly lucky in that the hospital I go to has three nurse counsellors and the one I see is a breast cancer specialist. She has visited me at home, phoned me frequently and it's very reassuring to know she's there and has the time to talk.

Because I coped publicly last time round I'm expected to

cope even better now. When people look at me sideways I feel I've got a label 'cancer' and I'm no longer Jill. It is hard enough trying to cope with it myself let alone having to cope with people feeling bad because they can't face up to me. I just wish more people would talk to me openly. One of the reasons why we've done this book is so that people will talk about it. It would help me and I hope it will help other women.

Jenny

Jenny has a 'horrific' family history of breast cancer. Almost all her female relatives on her father's side of the family have had it. She herself found a lump when she was 37, had a mastectomy and a week later an oopherectomy (removal of the ovaries). Since then she has had, as a precautionary measure, a course of hormone therapy. Jenny has three children, her first born when she was 30.

I first found a lump about the size of my little finger nail. We were on holiday (my husband had been working in Cyprus for six months and the children – aged three, five and seven – and I had gone to have a holiday with him). We had rented a house and we had been having a wonderul time. The horror of finding the lump was made even worse because we had been so happy. I had had a lump before when I was 21 which had been a small cyst but this time it felt different. I didn't tell my husband then. I didn't want to spoil the holiday – it was near the end – and he would have been so worried. I also felt if I told him it would make it more definite.

When we came home I told my husband and went to see my GP. He said he understood my concern but he wasn't too worried, but I could see in his eyes that he was very worried. He arranged for me to see a consultant the following Monday who said he thought it was cancer and that I should have surgery as soon as possible. I went to my sister's and wept on her kitchen table; then went home where my husband and I talked solidly.

We talked about the possibility of not having a mastectomy, but I really felt I wanted to get rid of it as soon as possible. I was terribly frightened. When I had been a medical social worker the breast cancer patients I had dealt with tended to be terminal and in great pain.

Q: Were you offered an alternative to mastectomy?

Jenny: No, the consultant said because of the area it was in and because it was a very fast-growing lump, mastectomy was the best treatment. In eight days the lump had grown from less than half an inch to two and a half in diameter.

Q: What kind of mastectomy did you have?

Jenny: I think it is called a modified radical. They took the lymph glands out because they were involved. Also this surgeon believes that women in their thirties (I was 37 at the time) should have oopherectomies (removal of the ovaries) following mastectomy. This was done a week after the first surgery. Personally this was more shattering because I wanted another child. I had my first child when I was 30 and I wanted another one. Then I broke down completely and my GP came to see me and insisted that the consultant talk to both my husband and I together and explain why it was necessary for my ovaries to be removed. He came to see us but rather reluctantly. A few years later I discussed this with him. He's a very quiet man and he feels the responsibility is with him and he knows best and that it complicates the issue if the patient gets too involved with what he wants to do.

I would have liked more time to discuss it. Nobody told me about the hot flushes that were going to occur. Nobody told me about the Mastectomy Association whilst I was in hospital – when they sent me out of hospital they told me to roll up my knickers and stuff them inside my bra! Because I feel so strongly about the lack of information available to me I am now involved with the Mastectomy Association and Cancer Link.

Q: When you left, did you have any kind of counselling?
Jenny: None whatsoever. The nursing care was very skilled,
adequate and totally unsympathetic. When I had the
second lot of surgery they even moved me from the room I
had been in and the nurses whom I knew to new faces in
the big ward. The only support I had was from my friends
and my husband who were marvellous. The new breast
care (counselling) nurses are now linking up patients with
the relevant voluntary organizations. I know a woman who
had a mastectomy with full support and she has come
through without all the bitter feelings that I obviously
have. Things have changed at that hospital, particularly
since I made it my business to complain to everyone whom
I thought was in a position to change the system.
Q: Were you relieved after the mastectomy?
Jenny: I don't know. I just assumed that the surgeon had
done the best thing for me and I must trust his judgement.
Q: Did you have any after-effects or other treatment?
Jenny: Artificial menopause – hot flushes, which I find very
hard to deal with. My GP tried me on Vitamin B6 for a
while. It's terribly embarrassing, particularly the face
because it's so obvious.
My family has quite a history of breast cancer, myself seven
years ago and recently my sister has had a mastectomy.
Also the last three generations of women on my father's
side of the family have all had breast cancer, and we have
all had mastectomies.
I went to a conference in Manchester. There was a
workshop on the side-effects of treatment, run by a lady
radiotherapist (who revealed toward the end of the session
that she too had had breast cancer). I told her of my
appalling family history and that I have three daughters.
We have all cut down on fats as it is thought to be one of
the contributory factors towards the disease. She said that
many studies have shown that it is not just diet but other
facts like the age for the onset of the menarche – periods –
and also the age at which you have your first child, the

view being that if you have your first child after the age of 25 you are much more likely to have breast cancer. My elder sister had had two children before she was 24 and she is the only one who has not had breast cancer. It's a dilemma now for women with career opportunities and not wanting to miss out on all sorts of things.

Q: How did you get involved in Cancer Link?

Jenny: Initially I saw an advertisement in the paper saying they were interested in setting up a local organization. As I was brought up in a small Scottish village I am a great believer in the strength and support a community can offer . . . I can see Cancer Link as a community-based support group.

Over the years I have become much more interested in what 'fringe' medicine has to offer. My sister and I had a discussion about visualization because she found the most difficult period was waiting for surgery.

If the same thing happened now I don't know if I would have a mastectomy or a lumpectomy. I have accepted the mastectomy but if it was the other breast I don't know. At least now I can stand in the mirror and look sideways and I have something . . . on one side.

Jo

Jo's mother died from cancer six weeks after having a mastectomy. Jo herself developed breast cancer. At 49 she had a lumpectomy and has a local recurrence in the same breast. She decided, following the lumpectomy, to have no further orthodox treatment and has since followed alternative therapies, finally choosing a Chinese therapy that involves acupuncture, dietary changes and other changes in life-style. She has no children.

I discovered a lump in my left breast and although my mother died of breast cancer I didn't go to the doctor for three or four months. I have a long history of bad health, steroids and numerous drugs. The doctor said she thought it felt like a lumpy breast and only to come back if it still bothered me. About nine months later I told some friends – one of whom had had breast cancer – and they insisted that I return to the hospital.

In the city I lived in at the time they had a walk-in clinic. I went there and saw a nurse who felt the lump and arranged a mammogram. Already I was beginning to feel that I was being taken over and because I wanted to be in control and I am also a photographer I took my camera and asked the radiographer to take a picture of the mammogram being done. This she did reluctantly. As the result of the test was suspicious I was then referred to a doctor. He told me not to worry, they were not absolutely certain what it was, but they would do a needle biopsy that morning. As the lump was quite big I would also probably have to go into the hospital and have it removed. He only vaguely mentioned the possibility that it might be breast cancer. I was given an appointment to go into hospital two weeks later. I had understood that I would be told the results of the tests as soon as possible but that was not the case. The other women and myself had a completely wasted day sitting around. The following morning we were all got ready for operation – exactly what we didn't know. It makes me very anxious to think about it even now. Suddenly a nurse came and pulled the curtains around me. She told me she was sorry, it was not the good news I had hoped for and the doctor would be round in a minute. I sat in bed crying, thinking, 'My God, she's just told me I've got cancer!' About half an hour later what looked like a child arrived at my bed – the older you get, the younger doctors look – accompanied by a retinue of white-coated figures. Their main object seemed to be to frighten me to death. We got off to a bad start because he couldn't seem to find a piece of paper that was vital to me and when I pointed out that he had the clipboard upside down he got offended. He then produced a pen and to my horror said, 'That's the breast that's coming off', and he put a cross on it. This was supposed to be a consultation with informed consent so I asked why I needed to have a mastectomy – what were the medical reasons? He couldn't tell me as he wasn't the consultant – who was busy operating downstairs – but I definitely needed surgery and it was essential that I sign a consent for operation as soon as possible. A nurse came back with the form and I refused to sign it until I had seen the consultant. She insisted he was terribly busy operating. I said my husband (the bloke I lived with but in this situation I had already learned you only have husbands) was on his way in and I wouldn't sign anything until I had talked to him. He arrived and gave me a great deal of support. I phoned everyone I could to find out my rights because at that time I didn't know what they were.

A nurse kept appearing with the consent form which I still refused to sign. I was still asking to see the consultant, but as he had gone to lunch it was impossible! They wanted to prepare me for the operating theatre immediately after lunch but I still insisted upon seeing the consultant. Finally this man rushed into the ward and up to my bed. He introduced himself as Professor X and asked me what the problem was and why was I refusing surgery. He refused to discuss anything with my boyfriend and insisted he leave the ward. Then the 'consultation' began. He could not seem to believe that I did not want a mastectomy. I told him that my mother had died six weeks after a mastectomy and if it was absolutely vital then I thought it could be done in stages. He said by not having a mastectomy I was endangering my health and anyway the mass may have moved. I said that if it had moved there was little point in mastectomy. He said he was worried it might settle on the chest wall. I said my worry that it might do this was greater than his, but no mastectomy. He then felt the lump and remarked on its size. At no time did he have my notes with him. Finally he capitulated and said I could have a lumpectomy instead. Little did I know that I didn't even have to have that either. So I signed the

form. As I was about to go into theatre a masked face
loomed out of the gloom at me and said he was going to do
the very best he could for me. I wondered if I hadn't
queried it whether his best would be enough.

So I had a lumpectomy and got back into the production
line. After several days they said I could go home but that
I would need to come back for radiotherapy. I agreed and
went home and waited to die. I was so depressed and I felt
so ill. Finally a friend suggested that I see a woman who is
an ex-nurse and is now a bereavement counsellor. She
helped me more than anyone else at that time. She had
worked for Professor X and finally she left because
although he was a brilliant surgeon his treatment of women
was inhuman. She also told me that we were in a trial area
and because I had refused mastectomy I would have
confused the computer figures. So what!

Four or five days later I received an appointment to have
a bone scan. Because I had been told nothing I thought it
was already in my bones. About a week later I returned to
out-patients for the results of the biopsies, which seemed to
have been temporarily mislaid. I had to sit stripped to the
waist in a windowless cubicle, with the hysteria mounting
around me. It was like waiting for the executioner to arrive
as the fear mounted in me. Finally the door was thrown
open and a beaming face informed me that the news was
good: it had not moved into the lymphatic system and all I
needed was radiotherapy. He was my neighbourhood
radiotherapist.

During this period I had been investigating the
possibilities of alternative treatment and I moved like
greased lightning. I went to the Bristol Centre and it was
like going from hell to heaven. They couldn't give me any
medical information because it was unethical, but they
listened and when I asked about the usefulness of
radiotherapy in my case they said that in their experience it
would not make a great deal of difference. I came away
determined not to have radiotherapy and also to move from

133

the provincial city where I had been living and back to London.

I went back to see my previous GP, the one who thought I just had a lumpy breast, and she said I absolutely must have a mastectomy and I was risking my life by refusing. She insisted I go and see Mr F. at a London teaching hospital and wrote a letter then and there. I opened it when I got home and it described me as 'this hysterical 49 year old woman whose mother died of breast cancer'. Not even any punctuation. I was enraged but I made an appointment to go back and see her. I realized that none of them know what anybody else is doing, there's such a time lag between letters. I told her I didn't like the hospital and I wished to be referred to a woman at another hospital. She grudgingly did this and I heard from that hospital that I could not see that woman as she was only involved in screening women and not post-operative patients. I had to go and see Mr F., the same one as at the other hospital. I conceded and finally saw God himself. He was basically a loving, benevolent, academic, patriarchal pig. Before he swept in with his entourage someone came in and went through a long questionnaire with me. When I said I was going to the Bristol Centre they didn't seem interested and anyway there was no space on the form for additional information. When Mr F. was questioning her about my history I interrupted and said I had not had three lumps removed, I had had three biopsies. He said the scars were far too big to be just biopsies. Thinking backwards, what they probably do in a trial area is to take out more than they need and put it into a flesh bank so various people can have a go at it. He said if I was his wife he would recommend a mastectomy and the scars would just break out in cancer if I didn't agree. I said I didn't want a mastectomy and so the discussion went on. He went to leave the room several times but each time returned with a new story to frighten me with. In the end he said he would get the radiotherapist to see me immediately, as there had now been a delay of about two months.

The radiotherapist was a very cheerful young man and arranged for me to start a course of treatment quickly. After I got home I decided I couldn't go through with it. I was following the regime Bristol had advised and I wanted to continue. The radiotherapy clinic rang me up and what seemed like a very sympathetic woman doctor arranged for me to come in and see her. I explained to her that I wanted to follow a naturopathic course and didn't want this to be interfered with by radiotherapy. She spoke to the head of the department and then asked if I would be averse to hormone therapy. I agreed to think about it but would first have to find out if there would be any interaction with my other treatment. The next day she rang me up and said that they had agreed I didn't need any further treatment. Next I had to see Mr F. again to find out the results of my various tests. They were all clear but he said he had got my records from the provincial hospital and in view of the type of tumour I had I *had* to have radiotherapy. I felt it was a very nasty game that was going on. I refused again but asked if I had jeopardized my chances of returning if it did break out again. He said that would not be the case but I would have to have an immediate mastectomy then. He was very upset and told me three of his patients had died as a result of going to the Bristol Centre.

I've learned from having had confrontations with two major breast specialists that they have a set routine they put you through in order to frighten you into treatment. It's like voodoo; if you don't do as you are told you will die. Mr F. also offered to replace my breast with a silicone implant after mastectomy. I have very large breasts and can't imagine a silicone implant slipping somewhere down my ribs, apart from the harm that can be done by putting it in.

This was my last brush with conventional medicine. I have never been back to the hospital or my GP. I continued with the Bristol regime, which was incredibly tight. I began to concentrate and feel much better than I

135

had done for years. My asthma, eczema and hay fever
vanished and I lost over four stone in weight. My libido
disappeared but has now come back when I fell in love
recently. The Bristol regime is basically all straight food:
no animal products, salt, sugar, coffee, alcohol or tobacco.
In Bristol one of the doctors is trained in Chinese medicine
and I told him I wanted to move towards this field. I found
a naturopath who started to treat me systematically, but
when she started on my back it packed up completely and I
was in agony. I didn't know what was happening but I was
too frightened to go back into the hospital. I read a lot and
spoke to lots of people and at one conference someone
suggested diagnosis by irridiology. I contacted an
irridiologist who discovered my eyes were a terrible mess
and that my lymphatic system was going mad. She
prescribed herbal treatment. Then my breast started to
swell up and a friend said that as my system was blocked
an acupuncturist would help. She gave me a name and I
contacted her. After two visits she suggested that I was
trying to ride two horses and that perhaps I would be
better adhering to just one regime like Chinese medicine
which consisted mainly of acupuncture, herbs, breathing
exercises and diet. I decided to switch to this. A large
tumour has recurred in my breast but I'm very happy with
what I'm doing. The aim is to dissolve the tumour with
herb sticks and localized heat. Cancer doesn't like heat. I
am also strengthening my immune system. I became
anaemic after my rigorous diet but now I have an almost
macrobiotic diet, white fish and meat and offal, which I get
from an organic butchers because of the very high hormone
content in ordinary meat. I have lots of rice and lentils and
soups but not lots of salads or cold food. I have no bread or
wheat gluten. I eat seaweed and sea vegetables. It's a great
diet and I'm enjoying food again.

I also decided that it was no good just working on my
body without healing my mind, so I am having therapy. It
is helping me to reconstruct myself.

I cannot at present do a full-time job and as alternative medicine has to be paid for my friends have put some money together to help pay for it. I spend far less on food than I used to. I have restructured my life completely. I used to be a workaholic and now I have veered towards gentle and therapeutic people. I announced that I was going to take two years out of my life and try to get better. I have been doing this for two years now and there was another year before when I had the lump. I am able to do this because I am a single person. My brother lives in Devon but he has his own problems. My mother died at 61 following a mastectomy six weeks before. It was said she died from secondary liver cancer. My father died three weeks after her. He just gave up.

I have no sentimental attitude to life. I think it's important to talk about suicide and euthanasia. People don't talk about it or anything else, which I discovered when I went to a women's therapy centre, where they had started a group for women with breast cancer. I sat there and came out with all these points. I had never done this before but if you have actually investigated the situation and are saying A, B and C are important but they are all still saying, 'Then I was in the waiting room', then you realize they have never really talked it through with anybody.

June

June is in her early 40s, is married with two young children and lives in London. She works part-time as a primary supply teacher.

When I first found a lump in my breast I went to the University Health Centre in Hong Kong, where we were temporarily living. They thought it was probably nothing but asked me to return in a month to review the situation. When I went back, they still thought it didn't have the

137

characteristics of a cancer, but as I was having a simple gynaecological procedure under general anaesthetic they suggested that they also looked at the breast lump and took a piece for biopsy. They also wanted to determine the nature of the lump with a frozen section.

There was another two-day delay and then I went into hospital. Partly because I knew Jill [Louw] I only signed agreement for removal of the lump, and said if it should turn out to be malignant I wanted time to make my own decision about mastectomy or alternative treatment. It was malignant and after I went home and talked extensively to a doctor, a woman who had had a mastectomy, and most of all, my husband, I decided to opt for surgery, as I thought this offered the best chance of survival. Also, because we were living in Hong Kong at the time and I have two very young children, the problems of lengthy treatment seemed insurmountable.

I don't regret the decision I made at the time. I had a semi-radical mastectomy quite quickly followed by a course of radiotherapy. At the end of our year in Hong Kong I had developed a cough which I thought was the cancer back again. Fortunately, a very nice English oncologist had just come to set up a new department and I went to see him. He gave me a lot of information and help and it was finally decided my cough was a result of radiotherapy, which had caused some lung fibrosis. I found the most distressing part of the entire illness was the radiotherapy. Not only was the actual treatment uncomfortable and debilitating, but the department staff were unhelpful and abrupt. I had no real counselling before but I did have some help from a woman who was trying to help people in my position. I didn't have a liver and bone scan before the operation, although I now understand this to be vital. I did have a bone scan after surgery which was clear. After our return to England I also had a liver scan and a chest x-ray.

My husband has been marvellous all the way through

and has supported and aided all my actions and decisions. I am so glad he was there.

We didn't try to hide anything from the children and their attitude has brought a note of humour into the whole business, particularly about the prosthesis. The first prosthesis was a very light affair and constantly rode up to my shoulder. Since we returned to London I have been supplied with a far superior model.

It's now a year since it all began and most aspects have become ordinary. I think I have come to terms with the situation, but I still have periods of anxiety and doubt.

Gladys

At the age of 48 Gladys had a mastectomy, breast cancer having been diagnosed. A year later it was found she had secondaries in her ribs and spine. She is being treated with hormone therapy (Tamoxifen) only and some of her secondaries have gone. She herself has also tried visualisation techniques to reduce the growth of the secondaries. Gladys has four children.

I remember saying if I ever had cancer I would want them to take anything they could as long as they left me able to fill the fridge and do the washing. If they had said this lump is malignant and you have a choice between lumpectomy and mastectomy it would have just thrown me into a quandary and I don't think I would have been able to make a more sensible decision. I had made my decision before in terms of my family, a husband and four children and I stood by that.

Q: Can we go back to when you first found a lump?

Gladys: Two years ago, I found a lump while I was in the bath. I didn't tell my husband until the next morning and I went to the doctor the same day. She phoned the hospital and I went a couple of days later. They were very quick and I went into hospital the following week for a biopsy. They told me before the biopsy they were pretty certain what it was because they could feel lumps under my arm as well.

Q: Could you feel the lumps under your arm?

Gladys: I didn't know about feeling lumps under my arm so I don't know. I could also tell by their reaction to the lump that they thought it was cancer. They also asked me to sign a form and told me if it was malignant that I would probably have to have radiotherapy. When I asked why, they said it was the safest way of ensuring that it did not travel.

I had a terrific distraction at this time because my third child was starting his O levels the day that I was having the operation and I was determined to show everybody that it made no difference at all. I also think both my husband and I were helped by the tremendous example of Lucy as someone who had got through it and was now in her fifth year.

Q: So you had a mastectomy?

Gladys: Yes. I didn't know it was malignant until afterwards but inside me I knew anyway. I was being treateed differently to other people I had known who had innocent breast lumps. I had said they could take the breast off if it was malignant, so it really wasn't such a shock to wake up and find it gone. The worst part came next, waiting for them to come and tell me if it had spread. Five days after the mastectomy they told me that the nodes were involved. I felt sorry for them having to tell me, it's such a difficult thing to get right; one sister said to me, 'Now you must live every day as it comes.' I thought I was going to die any minute. My husband was very good because he was very casual and said hundreds of women have breast cancer and to think of Lucy.

Later I asked the surgeon how I would know if it had travelled somewhere else, mainly because I had had a friend called Rita who had breast cancer which eventually went to the bone and she died. The surgeon said the bone involved would start aching. This was difficult for me as I

140

have had a bad back since the birth of my second child and I've got arthritis in the fifth vertebra or whatever, so every time I had a twinge of pain I thought of Rita. However, I was very optimistic for a year and I thought I had beaten it. In the summer the back ache got worse and I started to feel rotten. I tried to rationalize it. I am a nursery school teacher and bending over low tables does not do your back any good. I was tired and needed a holiday. On holiday I got worse so when we came back I insisted I have a bone scan, which for some reason they seemed reluctant to do. The bone scan showed that I had hot spots in my ribs and up and down my spine, much to the doctor's surprise. I felt much worse than before, it was a real smack in the face. They had taken my breast away and I thought that was the end of it. In spite of having radiotherapy afterwards it had still travelled to my bones. That seemed to me to be really sinister. They couldn't take my bones away.

Q: Did you have a bone scan before the mastectomy?

Gladys: No, there wasn't time.

Q: We would like each woman to have a bone and liver scan as a routine pre-operative check. Do you think this would enable you to think about alternative treatment?

Gladys: I didn't know about bone and liver scans, but now I think they should be done routinely. Also the hospital I first went to didn't have the facilities to do scans.

Q: Did you have problems with your arm after mastectomy?

Gladys: I had a lot of pain afterwards which I thought was part of the surgery, but I kept doing vigorous exercises until the pain was agonizing. Eventually I went back to the hospital for radiotherapy and I asked to see the physiotherapist. She stopped the exercises immediately and I had to put ice packs on my arm twice a day. I had an inflamed tendon which was being made worse by the movement. They said it was nothing to do with the mastectomy.

Q: What treatment are you having for the 'hot spots' in your spine and ribs?

Gladys: They put me on Tamoxifen straight away in
September. They also discovered I was badly anaemic,
which was probably why I had felt so dreadful. Now I am
pumping myself full of vitamins and iron and they have
made an enormous difference to the way I feel.

Q: Did they tell you what Tamoxifen is supposed to do and
do you have any side-effects? The manufacturers claim
there are virtually no side-effects but we are a bit sceptical.

Gladys: They said Tamoxifen was supposed to starve the body
of oestrogen, which breast cancer seems to feed on. They
also said they had some very good results, some secondaries
had disappeared altogether with this drug. Much to their
amazement I am still having periods, although I do get
some hot flushes. I have put on some weight and I get
these terribly itchy patches on my skin. I asked if I could
have another bone scan after a few months because
although I felt better I wanted to know if the hot spots had
altered. The pain was different from the arthritic pain I
had had for years, more a burning, almost like a humming
that got louder and softer. Now in my cheerful moments I
can almost convince myself that it was all arthritis.

Q: What has happened to the hot spots in your ribs?

Gladys: Initially they only told me about the areas in my spine
and it was only after the second bone scan that the ribs
were mentioned. I had been trying visualization, imagining
the Tamoxifen pills rolling up and down my spine. There
had been a marked improvement in my spine but another
hot spot had appeared on my ribs. After they told me about
the ribs I imagined the pills still rolling up and down my
spine, but when I got to my ribs I turned them on their
back and imagined them like a chamois leather shining my
ribs. I still do this frequently, but not as often as I should.
I wish they had told me earlier about the ribs.

Q: Have you made any dietary changes?

Gladys: I wrote to the Bristol Clinic and they sent me tapes
and literature. I have it on top of my wardrobe and I keep
it as a sort of insurance policy if ever the hot spots come

back. I haven't even opened it yet. After reading *The Gentle Way With Cancer* I followed a vegan diet for three days but it was impossible; it took much longer to buy and prepare food and my family didn't like it at all. At every meal I was eating different food to them and it was a constant reminder that I was ill. I didn't want it to dominate my life.

Q: After the mastectomy were you given a prosthesis, advice on exercises for your arm, the Mastectomy Association telephone number or any form of counselling?

Gladys: Because I was discharged rather quickly and there was nobody in the appliance department at the time a nurse and I went down and opened lots of boxes and I just pushed them into my bra until I found one that was right and comfortable. I was given no other advice or information. If I hadn't known someone else who had been through it I don't know how I would have managed. She was indispensable to me.

I have had no other treatment apart from Tamoxifen. The latest bone scan shows remarkable improvement. I take multi-vitamins and iron, but I have had a very poor response from doctors about the value of complementary medicine. When I asked about calcium tablets I was just told to eat more cheese, but I want to keep my weight down and not eat too much fat. I also no longer eat red meat. I wish they would take me seriously.

People have since asked me whether I would have liked a choice of treatment. I had already made a mental decision to have surgery and it would have been double agony for me to have had a biopsy and then to have to make another decision. Counselling would have been a great help.

Vivienne

Vivienne is in her forties, single and has no children. The only known case of breast cancer in her family is that of her mother's sister. Recently she had a mastectomy but has had no further

143

orthodox treatment. Vivienne however decided to follow a course of alternative treatment using the Bristol Centre's advice on diet and changes in life-style.

Cancer is such a scary idea to those who haven't got it that when I heard that a friend who is about the same age as me had cancer of the breast my first reaction was shock and horror. The second reaction was relief that so far I had avoided it, and to reassure myself I felt round my breasts, which was something I hadn't done for years. I immediately found a lump.

My response was to deny that I found anything but the next day I had another inspection and accepted that there was indeed a lump. After a virtually sleepless night I rang the doctor the next morning, a Saturday. The doctor on duty did not think there would be any point in seeing me as it would be too late to arrange an appointment at the local hospital breast clinic for the following Monday and anyway most lumps are not in fact malignant. I made an appointment with my own doctor for the following Tuesday, but the three intervening days were amongst the worst times of the whole experience because it was then I had to come to terms with the possibility of having cancer, and by the time I got to see my own doctor, I was sure that the lump was cancer. My doctor confirmed that there was a lump and arranged for me to go to the hospital the following Monday, doing her best to convince me that though she could not tell very much about the lump from an external examination it was more likely statistically to be benign than malignant. She also told me about the needle biopsy they would do. The next week was not so bad as I began to accept the possibility that it might not be cancer.

The surgeon who saw me at the hospital was wonderfully sympathetic. He asked me a number of questions including the date of my first period and whether any of my family had breast cancer. My mother's sister was undergoing treatment for breast cancer at that time but it had not

occurred that there might be a connection. The surgeon
said that there could be, and I immediately felt doomed.
However, he said that he was going to do a biopsy then
send me for an X-ray and he would have the result by the
time I came back. The needle biopsy was a bit painful,
although both the surgeon and the doctor said it wouldn't
be. The surgeon apologized for hurting me but wanted to
be sure that he got enough to give a clear result. He
explained that although there was a slight chance that the
result might be wrong, in 99 per cent of cases it gave an
accurate indication of whether the lump was malignant or
not. When I got back from X-ray he practically hugged me
and said it was definitely benign. I immediately forgot I
had ever been worried about it and when he said he
thought the lump should come out anyway I bargained
with him for as late a date as possible – two weeks away –
so that I could finish all I had to do before the Christmas
holidays.

In hospital a surgeon and his team of six examined me,
looked at the answers I had given to the first surgeon's
questionnaire and explained that he would like to do a
frozen section on the lump as soon as he had taken it out,
and if I wished I could sign a form which would allow him
to perform a mastectomy if the lump should turn out to be
malignant. I was very shocked. I asked him what the
chances were that it was likely to be malignant and he said
50–50, in spite of the biopsy report. I asked him what the
alternatives were and he said he could do a lumpectomy
and sew me up again, so that I had more time to think, but
that if the lump was malignant he would have to take a lot
anyway. I realized that what he was trying to tell me was
that since my breasts were so small and the lump was
under my nipple there would be nothing left anyway. I
asked if this was what he meant and he said he thought I
would be more satisfied with a straight scar. This was the
first time I had thought of what it would be like to lose a
breast. Even the problem of having cancer suddenly paled

into insignificance, and I wished all the seven sympathetic faces would just go away so that I could cry. The surgeon said he would come back in the morning and would answer any questions I had and I need not sign for anything until just before the pre-med. So I had a very different evening from the one I had planned, and it must rate as the worst time of the whole experience. Before going into hospital I had told friends not to visit me on the first evening. I had also told my doctor that the lump was definitely benign. Now I suddenly felt very alone. Luckily one of my friends disobeyed the visiting ban so I was able to talk things over with her and she helped me to think what questions to ask in the morning.

When I asked my questions I was answered in full and very sympathetically. The surgeons never volunteered any information but they always answered questions and never lied. I decided then that I had to have the operation because it seemed that otherwise I would never know whether I had cancer or not. So I went into the operating theatre not knowing what was going to happen to me and woke up with what they called a simple mastectomy, which was the removal of the breast and the gland under my arm. That day I struggled to be positive about it. Audre Lorde has described this struggle very well in the *Cancer Journals*. We all seem to think of the Amazons! There was no counselling in the hospital and I really needed it then. If anyone cried, Sister would come and tell you things would be all right, but I didn't cry so nobody came. There were four of us who had the operation at the same time so we counselled each other. Though the others had all had positive biopsies they were no less shocked after the operation. What surprised all of us was the weakening effect of the operation itself. I did not have much actual pain, except where a drain tube rubbed against a bone when I tried to lift my arm above my head. We dreaded visits from the physiotherapist, but in retrospect I am very grateful to her since I have not had any trouble with my arm in the year since the operation.

I had a lot of visits from friends, including my doctor who had somehow found out what had happened to me, and there were dozens of cards and bunches of flowers. All this recognition that something important had happened was very helpful to me.

My parents came as planned for Christmas and it did drain my energy a lot. But I think it was better to have them there than to have excluded them, and my father and my friends were very supportive, which was one of the nicer surprises of the event.

Two friends came up from England at New Year and took me back with them for a month. In their company I was able to cry and begin to take responsibility for healing myself. I read a lot of books about alternative treatments for cancer. After coming back to Glasgow for a check-up I visited the Cancer Help Centre in Bristol and went on their diet and took vitamin pills and slowly began to get some energy back. I also visited a homoeopathic doctor in Southampton, met Kit Mouat who is a living example of the efficacy of the 'gentle' treatment of cancer, and I decided that in future this was the way for me. The success rate of alternative treatment seemed at least as good as those of conventional treatment anyway and a lot less invasive. If I had known in the first place that I definitely had cancer, if I had known about alternative treatment as I know now, if it hadn't been Christmas and if I had realized how debilitating the operation is, I think I should not have let knives near me at all. On the other hand, since I did not know these things I do not regret what has happened. It turned out that I had cancer in my lymph nodes as well so they did not come out for nothing. And I know from the analysis that was done on them that my cancer would respond to hormone treatment, so there are some big guns there if I want them. My doctor, I think, would have liked me to have hormone treatment, but the hospital did not suggest it and both doctor and hospital are

147

happy to let me do things my way. My doctor prescribes the vitamins and minerals that the Bristol Centre suggest.

My energy is still not quite back to normal nearly a year later, but I was able to go back to work after Easter and do six weeks quite gruelling teaching in India in the summer. My morale is also quite good I think, although I can't help fearing that every ache is bone cancer, and I sometimes discover lumps that no one else can detect. I am also getting used to my asymmetrical shape, though I don't know whether I should have adapted so easily if I'd had larger breasts. The idea of flaunting the absence, as Audre Lorde at one time recommended, is abhorrent to me as it seems to invite a voyeurism that I do not want to be an object of. The things that I have always preferred to dress in are in any case fairly discreet about the number of breasts beneath them. I think my values and my life-style have changed more than my outward appearance. I rush about less, spend time on myself – which I always felt selfish about before – say what I think more, and am generally less worried about control and invasion. I am lucky enough to have a very good counsellor; I learned a little yoga in India; I have discovered that I have some very good friends, and by allowing myself to be dependent have paradoxically seemed to become more truly independent. In some ways having cancer has been a very liberating experience.

Hazel

Nine years ago, at the age of 41, Hazel had a radical mastectomy. She had no additional treatment following the surgery and has had no recurrence. Hazel married when she was 28, had two children in her early thirties and her marriage broke up about a year after her treatment for breast cancer.

It was nearly nine years ago now and I'd had a very bad spring – my father died, my children were ill, we moved

148

house, etc. One morning at half past seven I discovered a lump on the side of my left breast quite close to where it joins the body. I waited until surgery hours and rang the doctor. He thought it was connected with my period and told me to come back and he would reassess it. A week later it was the same so he referred me to a hospital, telling me he thought it might be a cyst. The hospital were almost as casual. The registrar told me that it was not very stuck to the wall, it was probably all right, but very casually thought they might just have to have me in 'to have a look'.

I told all my friends about the cyst I had to go into hospital to have removed in about ten days' time. Only one of them said that if it proved to be any more than that I would at least be in the right place, but I still insisted that it was only a cyst. My world fell apart when I went into hospital and spoke to a woman who was just about to have her second breast removed. When I asked her how she found out it was cancer she told me it was thought to have been a cyst! It literally did not occur to me until then that I might have breast cancer. I had a terrible night.

The next day I had a biopsy and when I woke up I had a large plaster across my breast. Then the waiting began. Each day I said, 'Anything?' and each day the answer was 'No.' Finally on the evening of the second day the surgeons came to see me and told me my biopsy proved to be malignant. I was distraught beyond measure and burst into floods of tears. The only thing that kept me going was my young children – my son was 11 and my daughter just 9. I felt if I could only survive long enough for them to reach maturity then I could manage to cope.

I asked the staff to tell my husband as I didn't feel I could. That night I had half a sleeping pill although I am anti most drugs. The next day I had a bone scan which was all right because a nursing friend of mine had come to see me and she was able to stay with me.

Q: Was the bone scan painful?

Hazel: No, it was an intravenous injection and then just laying under a machine going backwards and forwards over your body. The worst thing is the fear of what it might reveal.

Q: Did they do a liver scan?

Hazel: No. Only after reading afterwards that the liver is the most likely place for breast cancer to spread did I realize why they kept feeling down there (indicating liver region).

After lunch that day the consultant came and told me that he would do a radical mastectomy the following day. I was so terrified that I agreed; besides, I was given no choice. I think the radical was because the lump was so far round onto the chest wall (under the arm) and the radical took away the lymph nodes.

Q: Was there any involvement in the lymph nodes?

Hazel: No. That is actually one of my chief annoyances because I find the loss of that line there [indicating line from upper under arm to body] which I think is a beautiful line and the mucky armpit worried me more actually than the loss of the breast. As it transpired that it wasn't necessary I am surprised that they didn't take out a sample. There was *no* real discussion at all of alternatives; for example, not doing anything or the balance between a radical and a simple mastectomy. They didn't suggest radiotherapy and because of this I think I was at the time quite pleased to have the radical.

Q: Did they suggest just a lumpectomy?

Hazel: No. I think things have changed a lot in nine years. I had the surgery the next morning and don't remember much as I was pretty heavily drugged.

The following Friday there was an article in the *Guardian* which said that mastectomy was not necessarily the cure for breast cancer, there were all these other methods. I went mad that weekend. Apart from all the shock and trauma I was thinking that I possibly needn't have had it. Oh, that was a terrible weekend. My husband tried, but he couldn't cope with himself, let alone me. I could see a graveyard from the ward window and I thought I could see my mother's gravestone with my name written on it. I had

lots of friends and they were the people who gave me
terrific support, but there was no specific psychological
help from the hospital.

Q: Was any counselling offered?

Hazel: No, but five years later they offered to send me to a
psychiatrist or psychologist.

Q: Do you think that it would have been of benefit to you if
there had been a counsellor who dealt specifically with
breast cancer?

Hazel: I thought at the time that I coped with it all right.
Afterwards my GP was kind and helpful. Where I felt let
down was the Mastectomy Association, which I felt was a
toothless organization. I would have liked to have got
involved and I suggested . . . but they said they couldn't
have any meetings, they abided by their constitution. I felt
the Health Service appointed an organization regardless of
its usefulness.

Q: Do you feel there is indecent haste for surgery?

Hazel: Oh yes. If I had been living in a more natural and
relaxed relationship I might have found it earlier. But my
father was dying of cancer in Canada and I don't think my
husband and I had made love for two months. If we had
we might have found it earlier. I only found it by chance.
Then there was a delay of a few weeks but once you are in
hospital they have you by the short and curlies.

Two days before I was discharged my husband and I
went for a walk and we discussed what we were going to
tell his family. My mother-in-law was appalling and I
couldn't bear the idea of her coping with my cancer so I
had decided I did not want them to be told. I had made a
decision not to be put upon by anyone ever again – of
course that hasn't happened – but my husband couldn't see
what a state I was in and he said he would leave me and
would get a divorce. Although what I had said was the
truth I probably would not have said it had I not been at
such a low ebb.

Q: What was the relationship like before the mastectomy?

Hazel: He had become very reticent. I think the fact that we split up a year later and subsequently divorced was brought to a head because of the cancer, which was maybe a symptom of the strains of the marriage over the past 10 years. I have read somewhere that breast cancer seems to be prevalent among women who suppress their anger and repress their feelings.

Q: What was the sexual effect of having had a mastectomy? How did you deal with it?

Hazel: Not good, although strangely enough immediately after the operation my husband was a much better lover, for about six months. I never discovered why and it didn't last. I think it is for me a greater limiter of sex life. I have a lover who is a few years younger than me. The first time we made love I was very apprehensive but the second time we talked about it. He said I should warn people and perhaps consider an implant. He was very persuasive but there is no way I am going to have an implant because someone else wants me to have it. Also my husband and I never made love with the light on and I am very conscious of my body. Last time I kept my bra and prosthesis on but that is not really the solution. The answer is for somebody not to mind at all.

My attitude to breast jokes is markedly different from before. I am much more concerned about the effect of women who only have one breast. I have sometimes made myself quite unpopular with my outspokenness.

I was a 28-year-old virgin when I married, after being brought up in the repressive 1950s. I sometimes wonder whether breast cancer can be caused not just by having babies late but also years of repression.

Q: We're all appalled by disfigurement, aren't we?

Hazel: Yes, particularly because breasts are so much a part of sex. I'm 50 and I think my generation were taught to hate their breasts. As a teenager I remember thinking they were an embarrassment. There were no bras that fitted properly. Breasts symbolized growing up into the awful world of dreadful things. I wonder with the women's movement and (a) emancipation of attitude to their bodies and (b) being allowed to speak their minds, whether there is going to be as much breast cancer in the future. I think I am very much of the stress school, tremendous rows with my mother over school, church, inadequacy, and then later on a marriage which was not satisfactory. My husband had a nervous breakdown and far from offering support his family blamed me, so I just had to cope alone. Most women have a similar story.

Q: Do you live in fear that the cancer is going to recur?

Hazel: No, because I have had to get on and cope with my life and take charge of it myself. I made a resolution that I would not be bullied or taken advantage of again. With hindsight I should have split from my husband in the second, third or fourth year of marriage, but the old church teaching dies hard.

Q: After the mastectomy did they assure you that there would not be any recurrence?

Hazel: Yes. They said the chances were high because they had got it early. When I asked what the chances were they couldn't give me any exact facts because there weren't any available. I read somewhere that there are 25,000 mastectomies done a year. If that is possible there are hundreds of thousands of women going around the streets with only one breast. Last year I went to an open air Green gathering. In the women's tent there were a lot of people naked. It was a sunny day and the old people and the people who weren't beautiful looked beautiful. I broke down and cried and the people came up and comforted me and I told them my problem. One person said I hadn't mourned enough. There was never any opportunity to cry, I just had to be a good, young, bright thing and get on with my life. If I was married to someone who had had something so devastating I would try and build bridges and let them see that you knew to a certain extent what they had gone through. I came back from that gathering

153

determined not to wear a prosthesis. If we all did it we wouldn't have to pretend it had never happened.

The quality of the prostheses was bad in the beginning. They gave me this very light cap which rode up all the time. Their answer to that was a bit of elastic or sticky tape. There is a more expensive one with a bit of a hollow on the chest and a nipple which is the right weight and stays in place because of the suction, but it took me years to get this one. If you buy it they put VAT on, so you have to go to the doctor to get a piece of paper proving that you have had a mastectomy. When you show this to the shop you are exempt from VAT. As if anybody who hadn't had a mastectomy would go and spend £38 on a false boob, apart from Danny La Rue. When I complained to the Mastectomy Association they said some surgeons will give you nothing, but say you can go home and make your own out of bird-seed. That's no consolation.

Ann

Ann was 28 when she found a lump in her breast. Although she had age on her side, it took many weeks, much stress and painful treatment before the lump was finally removed and she was reassured it was not cancerous. She has two children, the first born when she was 25.

Q: What was your first symptom?
Ann: Well, I just felt a lump one day while I was having a bath. I ignored it for a few days because I was due for a period and I thought it might be connected with that, but after the period it was still there. A few weeks later my husband discovered it and asked why I didn't go to see the doctor. I said I was beginning to get a bit worried about it but I would leave it until after the next period and see if it might go then – which I didn't. Eventually, after about 10 weeks I think, I eventually plucked up the courage and went to the doctor.

Q: Why didn't you go to the doctor when you first found a lump?

Ann: Because I was frightened. The GP and his colleague examined the lump, discussed it in front of me – then said, 'I think you should see our breast surgeon, Dr H.' Well, then I started shaking, as soon as they said 'surgeon' I just imagined someone with a knife at the ready. My GP told me that she was a very good surgeon and that he would arrange an appointment as soon as possible. Two weeks later I went to the hospital and saw a young doctor, who asked me the same questions – Why hadn't I gone sooner? Was I worried about it? – and then he said he didn't think it was anything to worry about but he was going to book me in for a mammogram. I hadn't a clue what he was talking about and he didn't explain any further. About two weeks later I had a mammogram, which was not pleasant. I went back to the hospital a week later and the same doctor said the mammogram showed a lump – which I already knew. The next step was to remove some fluid from the lump, which they did a week later.

Q: Did they tell you what they were going to do?

Ann: They just said they were going to take a bit of fluid out to examine it under a microscope. I don't think I've ever felt anything as painful. They took quite a lot of fluid from the lump and told me to come back in a week. They still couldn't give me an answer, except to say that they thought there was some infection. They gave me a week's antibiotics and told me to come back the following week and see the breast surgeon – Dr H. She was very brisk and arranged immediately for me to be admitted the following Monday for removal of the lump.

Q: Did she explain anything?

Ann: I was only with her for about two minutes! She just said, 'We're going to whip the lump out, examine it, and you should know then!' I was admitted the following Monday to a local hospital, and after waiting half a day for a bed I was eventually examined by three doctors. They told me

155

that they would take me to theatre in the morning and remove a piece of the lump. That evening when my husband was visiting me they came back again and re-examined me. After a lot of whispering outside my curtains, one of them, a lady, came back to talk to me. She said that they were rather worried about the lump and they thought that it might be cancer. If it was cancer they would need to examine the lymph nodes to see if they were infected also. She wanted my consent to do all this with a frozen section and also start chemotherapy immediately if necessary. This was the first time anyone in all this time I had been going to the hospital had said that it might be anything other than just a simple breast lump. Chemotherapy meant cancer, I knew someone who had had it. I was also terrified that they would remove my breast. I was in a terrible state and so was my husband. After visiting ended, the ward sister took me into her office and tried to explain its effects. She also said that if I had started the treatment I would have to wear a skullcap to try to stop my hair from falling out too much. It was the worst night I have ever spent, in spite of the sleeping pills I was given.

I went to theatre at 8 a.m. the next morning and remember very little until I came round. The first thing I did was feel my head to see if I had a skullcap on. Later on one of the nurses said, 'You're OK. You haven't got cancer.' I was all knotted up inside and didn't even feel relief. Later the doctor came, looked at the wound and said everything was fine. I said it looked horrible to me and he said I should just be glad the result was OK and walked out. I just dissolved into tears and couldn't seem to stop.

My husband had phoned that morning, after a sleepless night, to ask what had happened and he was told I was fine and he could visit later. Nobody ever spoke to him about the possibility of cancer.

Q: Did you talk to anyone?

156

Ann: Only to Jill. I knew she had had breast cancer and would understand how I was feeling.

Q: Would it have helped if when you first went to the hospital there had been a nurse counsellor?

Ann: Yes, I would have been ever so grateful. Each appointment, after waiting for hours, I was quickly in and out. They seemed to always be busy. After about eight visits when I finally saw the surgeon I was told to come in for surgery in a few days. I think I would have preferred it if they had said that in the beginning.

Q: Was chemotheraphy explained to you?

Ann: No, not really. They told me more about the side-effects than what it was supposed to do. It was supposed to be a breast unit at the hospital I was sent to but it seemed to consist entirely of surgeons.

Q: Did you think of getting a second opinion?

Ann: I did think about it, but I didn't know how to go about it. Besides, my GP had said that this was the best possible place to go, and he had sent lots of people there and they had been treated really well.

Q: If you got another breast lump what would you do?

Ann: I certainly wouldn't want to go back there again. I suppose I'd have to go back to my GP and ask to be referred somewhere else.

Q: Were you given any sense of choice?

Ann: No. But as each time I went to the clinic I saw a different doctor I found it difficult to talk to them. I was frightened and confused, but nobody ever asked me how I felt. It was only the night before the surgery that anybody ever said that it might be anything than an innocent lump. The doctor told me afterwards that it was a very big lump which did look suspicious, but as breast cancer is very rare in women under 35 they were pleased to discover that it wasn't cancer. Nobody at any time talked about alternative treatment.

Q: Did you examine your breasts before you had a lump and do you now?

Ann: Before occasionally, now all the time. I've got a bit
    paranoid really.

Q: Did they tell you what it was?

Ann: They said it was infected milk ducts which probably
    arose from when I had breast-fed my son – three years
    previously. I didn't understand what that meant.

Q: Did they ever show you a section drawing of the breast –
    where and what milk ducts are?

Ann: No, they never showed me any picture or really
    explained how the breast functioned.

Q: Did you go back to the hospital for check-ups?

Ann: No, I went to the GP to have my stitches out. The
    hospital had given me a lot of dressings because the wound
    was discharging but nobody told me how to dress it for me.
    Do you dress it standing up or lying down? Finally my
    husband did it for me. Eventually because the wound was
    so painful I had to go back to the GP. He prescribed
    antibiotics because I had a wound infection. Finally it got
    better.

Q: Did you ever have to go back to the hospital?

Ann: No. They also never advised how to examine my breasts
    properly and regularly. I wonder if I'm susceptible to
    another lump or if I'm more liable to get breast cancer.
    Nothing was explained to me.

Q: How did you find out how to examine your breasts?

Ann: Through women's magazines. I now do it properly every
    month. Neither my husband or I could go through that
    again. We couldn't even talk about it.

Q: Do you think you could have talked about it if it was
    suspected bowel cancer?

Ann: Yes, I think that would have been different. At the first
    visit to my GP they said, 'Don't worry, they're not going to
    cut it off yet.' Cancer terrified me, but my real fear was
    having my breast removed.

Q: Why for women, why for you was the thought of having a
    breast removed so totally threatening?

Ann: I think I wouldn't have felt a woman again, sexually.

Q: Did you fear it would affect your relationship with your
husband?

Ann: Yes, definitely. Even now I am confused about what
happened. All the stuff I had read tells you to go the doctor
immediately. I didn't because I was frightened, then they
made me feel really guilty about leaving it for so long. And
then it was eight weeks before they got me into hospital. In
the end it was all a big rush – into hospital, get this lump
out – if it is cancer.

Sarah

Sarah was 37 when she discovered symptoms – nipple discharge
– of a breast disorder. She has had two pregnancies – the first
when she was 30 years of age. Apart from her sister who had
similar symptoms, as far as she knows there is no other history of
breast disorders in her family.

As I was painting the kitchen I became convinced my left
nipple was wet. I was so convinced I took my sweater off
and there on my bra was a small wet patch. Quickly,
having been used to expressing milk for my first baby, I
gently stroked my nipple with my forefinger and thumb. A
thick, sticky, white substance that looked like condensed
milk oozed from my nipple. I stood in the kitchen and
froze. My mind raced. Nipple discharge I had read
somewhere could be a sign of breast cancer, breast cancer
meant mastectomy and mastectomy was the unthinkable.
Leaving the paint brush wet, the radio on, the kitchen in
disarray I rushed upstairs to look frantically through my
bookshelves to see if I had anything on breast cancer. I had
nothing. I sat in the bedroom in total panic. Slowly my
panic subsided a little. I remembered that my sister had
had similar symptoms and so I phoned her. She asked me
in great detail about the discharge and asked more than
once had there been any blood in it. I said no. She
reassured me that discharge didn't necessarily mean cancer

159

and it hadn't in her case. She advised me to go to my GP straight away. There and then I made an appointment with my GP but had to wait several days before seeing him.

My appointment with my GP was functional. He examined me and referred me, without comment, for immediate investigation at my local London hospital with a breast unit. My first visit to the hospital, about ten days after seeing my GP, was equally functional. I was asked to strip to the waist, visually and physically examined and then asked if I could express any discharge. Of course sitting there, semi-naked watched by the doctor, a trainee doctor and a nurse trying to produce even the tiniest droplet of discharge was a struggle. I managed one droplet which they said they would send off to be tested. I was also told that they would like me to have a mammogram. The mammogram was an equally demeaning experience with one's breast laid out between two metal plates. The plates were cold, the squashing of my breast between them painful and throughout the procedure I tried to chat casually to conceal my fear.

Between the mammogram and the next appointment with the hospital, about two weeks, I felt fear mount in me. I kept trying to visualize myself without a breast. I wondered what one would look like without a breast. How important to me were my breasts? We didn't talk about it. Fortunately at that time I was working quite hard, but always at the back of my mind was this fear. Finally the day came for appointment. A friend of mine, Veronyka, came to the hospital with me. We sat in the waiting room, her trying to distract me and reassure me. My name was called. I went into the room to see the doctor. He told me, to my immense relief, that nothing was found to be amiss with my breast. I was given an appointment to return in three months. I was so relieved I didn't stop to ask any questions. All I could think was, 'It isn't cancer. I'm all right'.

During those three months I continued to get discharge

intermittently. I also got pain on the left side of my
breast. The pain came and went at no particular time and
was quite different from the general tenderness I feel
in my breasts just before a period. On my return visit
to the hospital, being a little calmer and having done a
bit of reading on the subject, I decided to ask what my
symptoms were. I particularly wanted to know if the
symptoms could be an indication of a pre-cancerous state.
My asking 'What was wrong with me?' elicited the
response that 'You really shouldn't worry, nothing is
wrong with you', and by implication it was clear that the
doctor thought I was a neurotic woman worrying about
nothing. Pathetically I said, 'Well, I'd just like to know',
and in response the doctor said that if I was really worried
they would make a big concession and see me again in
three months.

With no explanation and with my symptoms continuing,
I kept worrying. Something, I was sure, was not
functioning properly in my breast even if it wasn't cancer.
When a small tender lump suddenly appeared in my left
breast just by my nipple I decided I would get a second
opinion. Steeling myself I phoned and made another
appointment at my GP's surgery, this time asking to see
the woman doctor there. I told her why I had come and
what I wanted. She asked why had I come to see her and
not gone to my own GP in that practice. I said that I
wanted to see a woman doctor as a woman might
'understand'. Somewhat petulantly she asked me who I
wanted to see and I told her. Grudgingly she wrote a letter
for me referring me for a second opinion to the surgeon of
my choice. Before going to her I had done some consumer
research and had 'asked around' to find out which
consultant might offer a more sympathetic and informative
approach. Since there is no 'Good Breast Clinic Guide' like
there is the *Good Birth Guide* the only thing one can do is
'ask around'. Unlike childbirth it's much harder finding
people to ask. It's not just that far more women have

children but that women with breast cancer all too often don't want to talk about it.

My consumer research proved correct. The way I was treated at the second hospital was quite different from the first. I was given a thorough examination. After feeling my breasts the consultant asked, 'Have you ever had a rapid weight loss.' I said yes I had, from an illness I'd had about three years before. 'That would explain why your breasts are so nodular.' At least, I thought, someone has explained, which he went on to do, why my breasts are nodular. To that point no one had explained; all they'd done was to exclaim, 'You have nodular breasts.' I had begun to think I had freakish breasts, average in size but nodular inside. The consultant then told me that they really didn't know what caused my combination of symptoms. He said that at each clinic he would see on average about three women with symptoms like mine and that he could offer little explanation except to say they would almost certainly go at the menopause. To my question could the symptoms be pre-cancerous he told me there was no evidence that they were, though of course that was not to say that I would not develop breast cancer. After asking me about the amount of pain, discomfort and worry I had he offered me a choice of three forms of treatment, explaining the pros and cons of each. I could have surgery, but that, in his experience, was not usually very successful and that I would, as likely as not, return a year later with the same symptoms. I could have hormone treatment, but that had side effects, or we could just 'wait and see'. The lump had gone down by the time I saw him and he told me that if I had another lump which didn't go down in two weeks I should return immediately. Also if the colour or nature of the discharge changed I should return immediately. Indeed, if I had *anything* that caused me to worry about my breasts I should go back. With that assurance I opted to play the 'wait and see' game. Another lump suddenly appeared and was extremely tender, especially when my young daughter accidently elbowed me in the breast. It disappeared almost as fast as it had appeared. I still get minuscule amounts of discharge periodically, a little pain but I haven't had another lump.

Perhaps the consultant was more considerate of me knowing that I was obviously a 'discriminating consumer' since I'd gone for a second opinion. However, ironically, given my symptoms, the most reassuring thing he said was 'we don't know'. His admission of fallibility gave me far more confidence than all the assurances that I had previously had that 'it was all right'. Most importantly, though, I felt that I was being treated as an adult, intelligent person by not just having things explained to me but by being offered a choice of treatment with the pros and cons of each form of treatment. I'm still 'waiting and seeing' and hopefully that's all I'll be doing for years to come.

14. Glossary

Adenoma: a tumorous growth that is non-cancerous.

Axilla: the armpit.

Benign: medical term for a non-cancerous condition.

Biopsy: the removal of a small section of tissue for examination by a pathologist in the laboratory to establish a diagnosis. Biopsies can be done by operation (excisional) or by the use of a needle.

Carcinoma: a cancerous growth which in breast cancer occurs in the cells lining the ducts and lobules of the milk production system.

Carcinoma in situ (pre-invasive): a cancerous growth that is contained in its place of origin and has not spread.

Chemotherapy: the use of cytotoxic drugs either to stop rogue cancerous cells spreading from the breast or to control those that have.

Clinical examination: when a breast disorder patient is given a clinical examination, the doctor gives the patient a physical examination on which he or she will make an initial diagnosis.

Cyst: a small non-cancerous cavity filled with fluid.

Cytotoxic: (see *Chemotherapy*): the word means 'cell-poisoning.'

Endocrine or hormone therapy: a form of treatment used to control hormone activity when cancerous growths are suspected of being hormone dependent.

Frozen section: a small piece of tissue is removed whilst the patient is unconscious, is frozen and sent for immediate examination by a pathologist. It is then preserved for further examination.

Homoeopathic: a form of treatment based on treating a disease by tiny quantities of drugs that in healthy people would produce symptoms like those of the disease.

Hormone therapy: see *Endocrine*

Implant: an artificial substance, usually silicone gel, which is inserted into the breast cavity to replace the natural breast.

Invasive: a cancerous growth that has spread from the place of origin and invaded the surrounding normal tissues.

Lesion: a change in the function or appearance of an organ which is caused by disease.

Local recurrence: a cancerous growth that reappears where the first growth was.

Lumpectomy: the removal of the cancerous lump. Lumpectomies can vary greatly in size and therefore deformity is dependent on how much of the surrounding tissue is removed.

Lymph glands: these are glands (nodes) through which lymphatic fluid is purified – and then recycled into the blood. The lymph glands around the breast, particularly those in the armpit – can act both as a blocker of cancerous spread and as a channel through which cancerous cells can spread.

Lymphoedema: this may occur following surgical removal of some or all of the lymph nodes. The arm swells up because fluid cannot drain away through the lymphatic system.

Malignant: abnormal growths (cancer) that can spread locally and to other parts of the body.

Mammary gland: the breast.

Mammography: the X-ray examination of the breast.

Mastectomy: surgical removal of the breast.

Menopause: commonly referred to as the 'change of life', which is when a woman's periods stop and she is no longer able to have children.

Metastasis: the spread of cancerous cells from the site of the original (primary) growth to other parts of the body.

Mass: a swelling or lump.

Node positive: when one or more lymph nodes are found to be invaded by cancerous cells.

165

Oedema: a swelling caused by accumulating fluid.

Oopherectomy: the removal of the ovaries – either by surgery or radiation.

Pathology: the section of medicine which studies the causes and effects of various diseases including cancer.

Primary tumour: the original cancer before it has spread.

Prognosis: prediction about how a patient's disease will progress.

Prophylactic: precautionary measures taken to prevent disease.

Prosthesis: an artificial replacement for parts of the body. Used in this text to refer to artificial breast forms.

Radiographer: the technician who either takes X-rays for diagnosis or administers radiotherapeutic treatment.

Radiologist: the doctor who interprets X-rays.

Radiotherapist: the doctor who plans and prescribes treatment by radiotherapy.

Radiotherapy: treatment with X-rays.

Secondaries: cancerous growth(s) that occur in other parts of the body which have been caused by spread from the primary tumour.

Systemic: literally means the whole body system. Systemic treatment aims to attack cancer wherever it may be in the body.

Tumour: any abnormal swelling or growth that is of no use to the body. Tumours can either be cancerous or non-cancerous.

15. Complaints procedures

Complaining

If you have a complaint to make about the way you have been treated either by your GP or by any medical personnel at a hospital then you should contact your local Community Health Council. It exists to represent the interests of NHS patients. There is one council in each health district and you can find their address and telephone number either in the phone book or at a library.

Complaining is a complicated and lengthy procedure but the first thing to remember is you must register a complaint within *eight* weeks of whatever gave rise to the complaint. Your Community Health Council will advise you how to proceed, to whom you should write and what the stages of the procedure are. Since it can all take a very long time it is worth keeping a detailed record of every stage. Start by writing down the events which caused you to complain while they are fresh in your memory and keep a photocopy of all correspondence.

Few complainants wish to turn their complaint into a formal legal action. Few legal actions against the medical profession have ever been won. There is value in registering a complaint. If people don't register complaints, doctors can claim they have no knowledge of dissatisfaction among their patients. If enough complaints are made about a particular hospital, or section of that hospital, then there is hope they will be brought to the attention of those concerned and changes made.

Changing your general practitioner

For a variety of reasons you may wish to change your GP. One reason is that it may be a quicker and easier process than going through the complaints procedure. You have the right to change, but doing so is not always simple and straightforward. If you live in a rural area you may have little choice.

The procedure for changing is as follows:

1. Choose the GP to whom you wish to transfer. Asking around is the best way of finding out about GPs.
2. Having chosen, you have to get the agreement of the new doctor to take you on. You then either have to get your medical cards signed by your own GP saying that he or she 'agrees to the transfer' or if you can't face your own doctor you have to send your medical card with your new GP's name to the Family Practitioner Committee. The address of your local Family Practitioner Committee can be found either in the phone book or at a local library.

16. Useful addresses

Self-help, informational and support organizations

The following is a list of national organizations and their head offices. Many have local contact people and local groups. The list is by no means comprehensive, but is a good starting-point.

BACUP
121-3 Charterhouse Street
London ECIM 6AA
Administration: 01-608 1785
Cancer information service: 01-608 1661
Bacup was set up in 1985 to give information about all forms of cancer and 'to give emotional support and practical advice to cancer patients and their families about living with cancer and its treatment'. It hopes to act as an 'umbrella' organization providing, through leaflets, audio-visual materials and a regular newspaper, a range of advice, information and support.

CANCER LINK
46A Pentonville Road
London NI 9HF
01-835 2451
Cancer Link offers information and support. It has an information service which aims 'to provide information to people with cancer, their families, friends and carers'. The support offered through Cancer Link groups 'aims to bring together people with cancer, their families and friends to provide emotional support and local information'. To find out about a local Cancer Link group, contact their head office.

CARE – CANCER AFTERCARE AND REHABILITATION SOCIETY
Lodge Cottage
Church Lane
Timsbury, Bath BA3 ILF
0761-70731
Members of Care have all had cancer themselves and offer advice and support to people who have cancer. They publish a newsletter and arrange home visits to give practical advice, information and emotional support.

HEALTH EDUCATION COUNCIL
78 New Oxford Street
London WCIA IAH
01-637 1881
While the Health Education Council does much to publicize general health needs, the literature they publish on breast cancer (self-examination and the different treatments), though a useful starting-point, is probably not detailed enough for most women. Their publications are easily available from local health education departments as well as from the above address.

MARIE CURIE MEMORIAL FOUNDATION
28 Belgrave Square
London SW1 8QG
01-235 3325
The concern of the Marie Curie Memorial Foundation is primarily in providing a nationwide domiciliary service for cancer patients as well as a network of nursing homes. They also publish information about various types of cancer and run an advisory service.

MARRIAGE GUIDANCE COUNCIL
Herbert Gray College
Little Church Street
Rugby
Warwicks CV21 3AP
0788-73241

Trained counsellors help with any problem in marriage or personal relationships. Cancer frequently puts personal relationships under great stress. Local branches can be found in the telephone directory under 'Marriage Guidance Council'.

THE MASTECTOMY ASSOCIATION
26 Harrison Street
Kings Cross
London WC1H 8JC
01-837 0908
The Mastectomy Association gives information and support to women who have had mastectomies. They offer information 'about the different types of prostheses (breast forms) that are available, also bras and swimwear suitable for mastectomees and other more personal matters'. Through their Volunteer Helpers, 'each of whom has had a mastectomy and come to terms with it', they offer support to other women by visiting in hospital or at home any woman who has had a mastectomy and wishes to talk to someone else who has had the same experience.

NATIONAL SOCIETY FOR CANCER RELIEF
Michael Sobell House
30 Dorset Square
London NW1 6QL
01-402 8125
The main role of the National Society for Cancer Relief is to try to provide practical help, for example, paying heating bills, etc., for cancer patients. It has also established the Macmillan Homes for terminal cancer patients and a domiciliary care service which provides specially trained nurses to care for cancer patients at home.

WOMEN'S HEALTH INFORMATION CENTRE
52 Featherstone Street
London EC1
01-251 6580 or 01-251 6589

171

The Women's Health Information Centre aims to make information on women's health available to women. They are slowly building up a library on women's health and women's issues. Through them and the national register of women's health groups that they are compiling, it is possible to find out about different local health and self-help groups.

WOMEN'S NATIONAL CANCER CONTROL
CAMPAIGN
1 South Audley Street
London W1Y 5DQ
01–499 7532
As an organization, the Women's National Cancer Control Campaign has, since its formation in 1965, been campaigning 'to help women to overcome their fears about cancer and to take simple precautions which could well save their lives'. They provide a wide range of information about the need for early detection of breast cancer and the means by which to do it – breast self-examination. Leaflets, films and other information about breast self-examination are available from them.

Addresses of some alternative medical centres

Alternative therapies are many and various, some more appropriate and successful in treating certain conditions than others. For a complete list of addresses accompanied by explanations of the different therapies see *The Handbook of Complementary Medicine* by Stephen Fulder, published by Coronet. The following are just a few that may be of use to those who have had breast cancer.

BOURNEMOUTH CENTRE OF COMPLEMENTARY
MEDICINE
26 Sea Road
Boscombe
Bournemouth
Dorset
0202–36354

The Bournemouth Centre practises a range of alternative therapies for a variety of ailments. It also acts as a cancer help centre 'using the gentle, nutritional approach back to health'.

THE BRITISH ACUPUNCTURE ASSOCIATION AND REGISTER
34 Alderney Street
London SW1V 4EU
01–834 3353
As the name implies this association mainly uses acupuncture as a therapy combining traditional acupuncture with a Western medical approach. Through their register you can get hold of the names of practitioners.

BRITISH MEDICAL ACUPUNCTURE SOCIETY
5 Sunningfields Road
London NW4
The society represents the recognition of acupuncture within orthodox Western medicine. All its registered practitioners have orthodox medical qualifications.

BRITISH NATUROPATHIC AND OSTEOPATHIC ASSOCIATION
6 Netherall Gardens
London NW3 5RR
01–453 7830
Naturopathy is more a preventive form of therapy than a treatment. Like other natural therapies it is based on 'a system of treating human ailments which recognise that healing depends upon the vital curative force within the human organism'.

CANCER HEALTH CENTRE
Grove House
Cornwallis Grove
Bristol BS8 4PG
0272–743216
The Cancer Health Centre is known better to people as the

Bristol Centre. Its approach is holistic and is based on a total approach to cancer, involving diet, metabolic therapy, self-healing, psychotherapy and healing.

HOMOEOPATHIC DEVELOPMENT FOUNDATION
Harcourt House
19A Cavendish Square
London W1M 9AD
01–629 3205
Through the foundation and its information service you can find out not just more about homoeopathy but also get information on homoeopathic treatment. There are a few homoeopathic hospitals and clinics where you can get treatment as an out-patient and/or in-patient on the NHS. Homoeopathy is based on treating like with like.

17. Further reading

Personal experiences

Most autobiographies by women with breast cancer are more than autobiographies. While they recount personal experiences they also raise other wider issues about treatments, social and medical attitudes.

Graham, Jory, *In the Company of Others*, Victor Gollancz, London, 1983.
Kidman, Brenda, *A Gentle Way With Cancer*, Century Publishing Company, London, 1985.
Kushner, Rose, *Breast Cancer: A Personal History and an Investigative Report*, Harcourt, New York, 1979.
Lorde, Audre, *The Cancer Journals*, Sheba, London, 1985.
Rollin, Betty, *First You Cry*, Signet, New York, 1977.

General books

The following is a list of books about breast cancer, its treatments, orthodox and alternative, the ethical issues that arise out of medical practice and books on the breast and cancer in general.

Bishop, Beata, *A Time to Heal*, Severn House, London, 1985.
Baum, Michael, *Breast Cancer: The Facts*, Oxford University Press, Oxford, 1981.
Faulder, Carolyn, *Breast Cancer*, Virago, London, 1982.
Faulder, Carolyn, *Whose Baby Is It?*, Virago, London, 1985.

Smedley, Howard, Sikora, Karel and Stepney, Rob, *Cancer*, Basil Blackwell, Oxford, 1985.

Milan, Albert, *Breast Self-Examination*, Liberty Publishing Company, New York, 1980.

Mouat, Kit, *Fighting For Our Lives*, Heretic Books, 1984.

Stanway, Andrew and Stanway, Penny, *The Breast*, Granada Publishing 1982.